Pediatric Nursing Today:

Current Trends and Best Practices with a Holistic Approach for Learning

DISCLAIMER

Introduction

A subspecialty of nursing known as pediatric nursing is concerned with pediatrics and the medical treatment of young patients up to adolescence. This is a crucial area of study since children's health differs from adults' due to the growth and development that takes place during childhood.

It is worth noting that certification as a pediatric nurse is not required to work as a nurse for children. However, obtaining specialized knowledge and training helps to improve job prospects and is recommended for nurses who have a passion for caring for children.

Typically, pediatric nurses collaborate with other medical specialists in a multidisciplinary team to give kids the best care possible. They are crucial in keeping an eye on the well-being of young patients and offering them support and care as they undergo therapy.

They may give immunizations or childhood vaccinations and ensure that kids follow their immunization schedule. A pediatric nurse also explains the children's health and the stages of treatment to the youngsters and their families.

A pediatric nurse may instruct and manage children's health care for members of the public or other medical professionals. Additionally, they can support clinical studies about frequent health issues affecting children and suitable treatment approaches.

It encompasses a wide range of topics related to the health and well-being of young individuals.

Chapter 1

Child Growth and Development

Child growth and development is a critical aspect of pediatric nursing, as it provides the foundation for understanding the unique needs and characteristics of children at different stages of their lives. Here are key points related to child growth and development in the context of pediatric nursing:

1. **Infant Development:**
   - **Physical Development:** Monitoring weight gain, height, head circumference, and motor skills.
   - **Cognitive Development:** Recognizing sensory and perceptual development, and object permanence.
   - **Social and Emotional Development:** Attachment, bonding, and emotional responsiveness.
2. **Toddler and Preschooler Development:**
   - **Physical Development:** Gross and fine motor skills, toilet training.
   - **Cognitive Development:** Language acquisition, preoperational thought, imagination.
   - **Social and Emotional Development:** Independence, socialization, peer interactions.
3. **School-Age Child Development:**
   - **Physical Development:** Continued growth, and development of permanent teeth.
   - **Cognitive Development:** Concrete operational thought, and academic skills.
   - **Social and Emotional Development:** Formation of friendships, and self-esteem.
4. **Adolescent Development:**

- **Physical Development:** Puberty, sexual maturity, growth spurts.
- **Cognitive Development:** Abstract thinking, decision-making.
- **Social and Emotional Development:** Identity formation, peer relationships, independence.

5. **Developmental Milestones:**
   - Understanding and assessing age-appropriate developmental milestones.
   - Recognizing variations in individual development.

6. **Developmental Assessments:**
   - Using standardized tools to assess developmental progress.
   - Identifying potential developmental delays and early intervention.

7. **Cultural Influences on Development:**
   - Recognizing the impact of cultural background on child-rearing practices.
   - Providing culturally sensitive care.

8. **Play and Development:**
   - Understanding the role of play in cognitive, social, and emotional development.
   - Encouraging age-appropriate play activities.

9. **Environmental Influences:**
   - Considering the impact of the physical and social environment on development.
   - Identifying and addressing environmental risk factors.

10. **Supporting Families in Understanding Development:**
    - Educating parents and caregivers about normal developmental stages.
    - Guiding age-appropriate activities and

interventions.

11. **Promoting Developmental Health:**
    - Emphasizing the importance of nutrition, exercise, and a safe environment.
    - Collaborating with other healthcare professionals for comprehensive care.

Understanding child growth and development is fundamental for pediatric nurses to provide age-appropriate care, identify deviations from typical development, and support families in nurturing their children's well-being. Regular assessments and ongoing monitoring are crucial components of pediatric nursing practice in this regard.

Physical, Cognitive, and Emotional Development Milestones

Child development encompasses physical, cognitive, and emotional domains. Here are some general milestones in each of these areas. Keep in mind that these are approximate guidelines, and individual children may reach these milestones at different rates.

Physical Development Milestones:

Infancy (0-12 months):

- Lifts head and chest when lying on stomach (around 2-4 months).
- Rolls over (around 4-6 months).
- Sits without support (around 6-8 months).
- Crawls (around 6-10 months).
- Pulls up to stand and stands with support (around 8-12 months).

Toddlerhood (1-3 years):

- Walks independently (around 12-15 months).
- Climbs stairs with assistance (around 18-24 months).
- Runs and jumps (around 2 years).
- Throws and kicks a ball (around 2-3 years).
- Begins to use utensils for self-feeding (around 2-3 years).

Preschool (3-6 years):

- Hops and stands on one foot (around 3-4 years).
- Pedals a tricycle (around 3-4 years).
- Catches a ball with hands (around 4-5 years).
- Ties shoelaces (around 5-6 years).
- Demonstrates hand dominance (right or left-handedness).

School-Age (6-12 years):

- Refines motor skills (e.g., improved handwriting).
- Develop coordination and balance.
- Experiences growth spurts during puberty.
- Engages in organized sports and physical activities.

Adolescence (12-18 years):

- Achieves peak physical growth during puberty.
- Develop muscle mass and bone density.
- Refines motor skills and coordination.
- Experiences changes in body composition and sexual maturation.

Cognitive Development Milestones:
Infancy (0-12 months):

- Respond to visual and auditory stimuli.
- Begins to explore objects with hands and mouth.
- Develops object permanence (understands that objects exist even when not seen).

Toddlerhood (1-3 years):

- Engages in parallel play.
- Shows interest in simple puzzles and stacking blocks.
- Learns basic cause-and-effect relationships.

Preschool (3-6 years):

- Develop preoperational thought (egocentrism, symbolic play).
- Expands vocabulary and language skills.
- Begins to understand concepts of time and space.

School-Age (6-12 years):

- Develops concrete operational thought (logical reasoning).
- Advances in reading, writing, and mathematical skills.
- Shows increased ability for abstract thinking.

Adolescence (12-18 years):

- Develop abstract thinking and hypothetical reasoning.
- Form personal identity and values.
- Prepares for higher-level cognitive tasks, such as critical thinking.

Emotional Development Milestones:
Infancy (0-12 months):

- Forms attachments and bonds with caregivers.
- Displays basic emotions (happiness, sadness, anger).

Toddlerhood (1-3 years):

- Experiences increased independence and autonomy.
- Demonstrates a wider range of emotions.
- Begins to understand and express emotions verbally.

Preschool (3-6 years):

- Develop empathy and understanding of others' emotions.
- Engages in cooperative play.
- Experiences emotional regulation challenges.

School-Age (6-12 years):

- Forms friendships and peer relationships.
- Develop a sense of self-esteem and competence.
- Begins to understand and manage more complex emotions.

Adolescence (12-18 years):

- Experiences increased emotional intensity.

- Forms deeper relationships outside the family.
- Navigates identity formation and self-discovery.

Understanding these milestones helps healthcare professionals, including pediatric nurses, monitor and support children's overall development. It also provides a framework for identifying potential concerns or delays that may require further assessment or intervention.

Age-Appropriate Assessments and Interventions

Age-appropriate assessments and interventions are crucial components of pediatric nursing, ensuring that care aligns with the developmental stage and individual needs of the child. Here are some general guidelines for age-appropriate assessments and interventions across different stages of childhood:

Infancy (0-12 months):

Assessments:

1. **Physical Assessment:**
    - Weight, length, and head circumference measurements.
    - Developmental milestones (e.g., motor skills, reflexes).
    - Growth charts for tracking development.

2. **Feeding and Nutrition:**
    - Assess breastfeeding or formula feeding.
    - Monitor weight gain and feeding patterns.
    - Introduce complementary foods at appropriate times.

3. **Sleep Patterns:**
    - Assess sleep duration and patterns.
    - Guide safe sleep practices.

Interventions:

1. **Immunizations:**
    - Administer vaccines per the recommended schedule.
    - Educate parents on the importance of vaccinations.

2. **Parental Education:**
    - Guide infant care and safety.

- Teach parents about developmental milestones.
3. **Support for New Parents:**
    - Address postpartum concerns and emotions.
    - Encourage bonding and attachment.

Toddlerhood (1-3 years):
Assessments:

1. **Developmental Screening:**
    - Evaluate gross and fine motor skills.
    - Assess language development and social interactions.
2. **Safety Assessments:**
    - Identify potential hazards in the home.
    - Discuss injury prevention strategies.
3. **Nutrition and Growth:**
    - Monitor growth and weight.
    - Assess eating habits and introduce a balanced diet.

Interventions:

1. **Developmental Stimulation:**
    - Encourage age-appropriate play and exploration.
    - Recommend toys that support fine and gross motor skills.
2. **Parental Guidance:**
    - Guide discipline and setting limits.
    - Offer support for toilet training.
3. **Immunizations:**
    - Ensure adherence to the vaccination schedule.

Preschool (3-6 years):
Assessments:

1. **Cognitive and Behavioral Assessments:**

- Evaluate cognitive development and school readiness.
- Screen for behavioral or attention issues.

2. **Vision and Hearing Screening:**
   - Conduct routine vision and hearing checks.
   - Address any identified issues promptly.

3. **Social and Emotional Assessment:**
   - Monitor social interactions and emotional well-being.
   - Identify signs of stress or adjustment difficulties.

Interventions:

1. **Early Education Support:**
   - Encourage age-appropriate learning activities.
   - Support readiness for school.

2. **Behavioral Guidance:**
   - Provide strategies for positive discipline.
   - Offer guidance on peer interactions.

3. **Family-Centered Care:**
   - Involve parents in the child's education and development.
   - Foster communication between parents and educators.

School-Age (6-12 years):
Assessments:

1. **Academic Performance:**
   - Monitor academic achievements and challenges.
   - Screen for learning disabilities if needed.

2. **Psychosocial Assessments:**
   - Assess social relationships and peer interactions.
   - Screen for signs of bullying or emotional difficulties.

3. **Health and Wellness Assessments:**
   - Check for scoliosis and other physical health concerns.
   - Promote a healthy lifestyle and nutrition.

Interventions:

1. **Educational Support:**
   - Collaborate with school professionals for academic support.
   - Advocate for any necessary accommodations.
2. **Health Promotion:**
   - Encourage physical activity and a balanced diet.
   - Discuss the risks of substance use and provide education.
3. **Counseling Support:**
   - Offer counseling for emotional and behavioral challenges.
   - Involve parents in the intervention process.

Adolescence (12-18 years):
Assessments:

1. **Psychosocial Assessment:**
   - Explore identity formation and self-esteem.
   - Screen for signs of depression, anxiety, or other mental health concerns.
2. **Sexual Health Assessment:**
   - Discuss puberty, sexual development, and contraception.
   - Provide education on sexually transmitted infections.
3. **Risk Behavior Assessment:**
   - Assess risk behaviors (e.g., substance use, risky sexual

behavior).
- ○ Screen for signs of self-harm or suicidal ideation.

Interventions:

1. **Health Education:**
   - ○ Educate on healthy lifestyle choices and self-care.
   - ○ Discuss the importance of mental health and stress management.
2. **Support for Independence:**
   - ○ Encourage autonomy and decision-making.
   - ○ Discuss future goals and career aspirations.
3. **Counseling and Mental Health Support:**
   - ○ Provide access to counseling services.
   - ○ Involve parents or guardians as needed for support.
4. **Educational and Career Guidance:**
   - ○ Assist with educational and career planning.
   - ○ Collaborate with school counselors and parents.

Age-appropriate assessments and interventions in pediatric nursing require a holistic and individualized approach. Regular communication with parents or caregivers is essential to ensure continuity of care and address any concerns promptly. Additionally, interdisciplinary collaboration with educators, mental health professionals, and other healthcare providers is valuable in supporting the overall well-being of the child.

Chapter 2

Pediatric Assessment

Pediatric assessment involves systematically gathering information about a child's health status through a combination of observation, interview, and physical examination. It is a critical aspect of pediatric nursing, helping healthcare professionals identify normal growth and development, detect deviations from the expected, and plan appropriate care. Here's an overview of the key components of pediatric assessment:

1. Health History:

- Obtain a thorough health history from parents or caregivers.
- Include information on prenatal and birth history, family medical history, and current health concerns.

2. Developmental Assessment:

- Evaluate age-appropriate developmental milestones.
- Assess gross and fine motor skills, language development, and cognitive abilities.

3. Nutritional Assessment:

- Gather information on the child's dietary habits.
- Assess growth patterns, weight gain, and any nutritional concerns.

4. Immunization Status:

- Verify the child's immunization records.
- Ensure that the child is up-to-date on vaccinations according to the recommended schedule.

5. Physical Examination:

- Conduct a head-to-toe physical examination.

- Assess vital signs, general appearance, skin, eyes, ears, nose, throat, chest, abdomen, musculoskeletal system, and neurological status.

6. Assessment of Systems:

- **Cardiovascular System:** Assess heart rate, rhythm, and peripheral perfusion.
- **Respiratory System:** Evaluate respiratory rate, effort, and breath sounds.
- **Gastrointestinal System:** Check for any issues with feeding, digestion, or elimination.
- **Genitourinary System:** Assess urinary output, genitalia, and signs of any urinary or reproductive concerns.
- **Neurological System:** Evaluate the level of consciousness, reflexes, and neurological responses.

7. Vision and Hearing Screening:

- Perform age-appropriate vision and hearing screenings.
- Refer for more comprehensive assessments if any concerns arise.

8. Psychosocial Assessment:

- Evaluate the child's emotional and mental well-being.
- Screen for signs of anxiety, depression, or behavioral issues.

9. Pain Assessment:

- Use age-appropriate pain assessment tools.
- Consider non-verbal cues for younger children and self-report for older children.

10. Family and Environmental Assessment:

- Consider the family's dynamics and support system.
- Assess the child's living conditions and any environmental factors that may impact health.

11. Cultural Competence:

- Consider cultural factors that may influence health practices and beliefs.
- Provide culturally sensitive care and respect family values.

12. Safety Assessment:

- Evaluate the child's home environment for safety.
- Discuss injury prevention strategies with parents or caregivers.

13. Laboratory and Diagnostic Tests:

- Order or perform any necessary laboratory tests or diagnostic procedures.
- Interpret results in the context of the child's health status.

14. Communication and Interaction:

- Communicate effectively with the child, adapting to their developmental level.
- Collaborate with parents or caregivers, providing education and addressing concerns.

15. Documentation:

- Record assessment findings accurately and thoroughly.
- Document any deviations from normal and the plan of care.

16. Follow-up and Monitoring:

- Establish a plan for follow-up care and monitoring.
- Coordinate with other healthcare professionals involved in the child's care.

Pediatric assessment requires a comprehensive and holistic approach, considering the unique needs and developmental stages of children. Continuous communication with the child and their family is essential for building trust and ensuring effective care. Additionally, pediatric nurses should stay updated on current guidelines and best practices in pediatric assessment.

Techniques for Assessing the Health Status of Children

Assessing the health status of children involves a combination of techniques that take into account their developmental stages, communication abilities, and the unique aspects of pediatric care. Here are some key techniques for pediatric health assessment:

1. Observation:

- **General Appearance:** Observe the child's posture, behavior, and overall demeanor.
- **Skin:** Check for color, temperature, texture, and any signs of rashes or lesions.
- **Breathing Pattern:** Observe respiratory rate, depth, and effort.

2. Interviewing and Communication:

- **Child-Centered Communication:** Tailor communication to the child's age and developmental level.
- **Open-Ended Questions:** Use open-ended questions to encourage children to express themselves.
- **Play-Based Communication:** For younger children, incorporate play to understand their feelings and experiences.

3. Vital Signs:

- **Temperature:** Measure using appropriate methods (oral, axillary, tympanic, or rectal).
- **Pulse:** Assess heart rate and rhythm.
- **Respiration:** Count respiratory rate, and observe for any signs of distress.
- **Blood Pressure:** Depending on the child's age and size, use an age-appropriate cuff size.

4. Developmental Assessment:

- Use age-appropriate tools to assess developmental milestones.
- Observe motor skills, language development, and cognitive abilities.

5. Physical Examination:

- Perform a head-to-toe examination, adapting to the child's comfort level.

- Use distraction techniques or involve parents to ease anxiety.

6. Growth Measurements:

- Record height, weight, and head circumference for infants and young children.
- Plot measurements on growth charts to assess trends.

7. Pain Assessment:

- Use age-appropriate pain scales.
- Consider the child's ability to self-report or use behavioral indicators for younger children.

8. Vision and Hearing Screening:

- Use age-appropriate vision charts and hearing tests.
- Refer for more comprehensive assessments if needed.

9. Laboratory Tests:

- Collect blood, urine, or other specimens as needed.
- Ensure proper preparation and communication with the child.

10. Dental Assessment:

- Inspect the oral cavity for signs of dental health issues.
- Provide education on oral hygiene practices.

11. Functional Assessment:

- Assess activities of daily living (ADLs) appropriate for the child's age.
- Consider any limitations or challenges in self-care.

12. Psychosocial Assessment:

- Evaluate the child's emotional well-being and mental health.
- Screen for signs of stress, anxiety, or depression.

13. Cultural Competence:

- Consider cultural beliefs and practices that may impact health.
- Adapt assessment techniques to respect cultural norms.

14. Environmental Assessment:

- Evaluate the child's living conditions for safety and health hazards.
- Discuss any environmental concerns with parents or caregivers.

15. Family Engagement:

- Involve parents or caregivers in the assessment process.
- Gather information on family dynamics and support systems.

16. Collaboration with Interdisciplinary Team:

- Communicate and collaborate with other healthcare professionals involved in the child's care.
- Share assessment findings and contribute to the overall care plan.

17. Documentation:

- Document assessment findings accurately and comprehensively.
- Include information on the child's response to interventions.

18. Follow-Up and Education:

- Establish a plan for follow-up care and monitoring.
- Provide education to parents and caregivers on maintaining

the child's health.

Adapting assessment techniques to the child's age, developmental stage, and communication abilities is essential in pediatric nursing. A holistic and family-centered approach ensures that the child's physical, emotional, and social well-being is addressed comprehensively.

Vital Signs, Developmental Screenings, and Physical Examinations

Vital signs, developmental screenings, and physical examinations are fundamental components of pediatric nursing assessments. These assessments provide valuable information about a child's health status, growth, and developmental milestones. Here's an overview of each:

1. Vital Signs:

Vital signs are key indicators of a child's physiological status. They include:

a. Temperature:

- **Methods:** Oral, axillary, tympanic, or rectal based on the child's age and cooperation.
- **Normal Range:** 97.8–99.1°F (36.5–37.3°C) for oral, 98.6–100.6°F (37–38.1°C) for rectal.

b. Heart Rate (Pulse):

- **Methods:** Count the pulse at the radial or apical site.
- **Normal Range:** Newborns (120-160 bpm), Infants (100-160 bpm), Toddlers (90-150 bpm), Preschoolers (80-140 bpm), School-age (75-120 bpm), Adolescents (60-100 bpm).

c. Respiratory Rate:

- **Methods:** Observe chest or abdominal movements.
- **Normal Range:** Newborns (30-60 breaths per minute), Infants (25-40 bpm), Toddlers (20-30 bpm), Preschoolers (20-30 bpm), School-age (16-22 bpm), Adolescents (12-18 bpm).

d. Blood Pressure:

- **Methods:** Use age-appropriate cuff sizes and techniques.
- **Normal Range:** Varies by age and height; refer to pediatric blood pressure charts.

2. Developmental Screenings:

Developmental screenings assess a child's milestones and achievements at different stages of growth. They help identify any potential delays or concerns. Screening tools include:

a. Denver Developmental Screening Test (DDST):

- Screens for gross and fine motor skills, socialization, language, and adaptive behavior.

b. Ages and Stages Questionnaires (ASQ):

- Assesses communication, gross and fine motor skills, problem-solving, and personal-social skills.

c. Modified Checklist for Autism in Toddlers (M-CHAT):

- Screens for early signs of autism spectrum disorders.

d. Pediatric Symptom Checklist (PSC):

- Screens for emotional and behavioral issues in children.

3. Physical Examinations:

A comprehensive physical examination involves a head-to-toe assessment. Key components include:

a. General Appearance:

- Evaluate overall health, alertness, and level of distress.

b. Skin:

- Inspect for color, texture, lesions, or rashes.

c. Eyes:

- Assess visual acuity, eye movements, and signs of any abnormalities.

d. Ears:

- Inspect for signs of infection or hearing issues.

e. Nose and Throat:

- Check for congestion, discharge, or tonsillar enlargement.

f. Chest and Lungs:

- Auscultate breath sounds and assess respiratory effort.

g. Cardiovascular System:

- Assess heart rate, rhythm, and peripheral pulses.

h. Abdomen:

- Palpate for tenderness, organ enlargement, or masses.

i. Musculoskeletal System:

- Evaluate joint range of motion, muscle strength, and posture.

j. Neurological Assessment:

- Assess the level of consciousness, reflexes, and coordination.

k. Genitourinary System:

- Inspect genitalia, assess urinary output, and evaluate for signs of urinary issues.

l. Growth Measurements:

- Measure height, weight, and head circumference (for infants).

m. Dental Examination:

- Inspect the oral cavity for signs of dental health issues.

n. Behavioral and Psychosocial Assessment:

- Observe for signs of stress, anxiety, or behavioral concerns.

o. Review of Systems:

- Systematically inquire about symptoms related to various body systems.

Tips for Pediatric Examinations:

- **Use Distraction Techniques:** Employ age-appropriate distraction techniques to ease anxiety.
- **Involve Parents:** Encourage parents to be present and provide comfort during the examination.
- **Communicate Clearly:** Explain procedures in simple terms and use play when appropriate.
- **Respect Modesty:** Ensure privacy and maintain the child's comfort and dignity.

Pediatric nurses must adapt these assessments to the child's age, developmental level, and individual needs, ensuring a holistic understanding of the child's health status. Regular screenings and examinations help detect potential issues early and contribute to the overall well-being of the child.

Chapter 3

Common Pediatric Illnesses

Pediatric illnesses can vary widely and may include infectious diseases, chronic conditions, and acute illnesses. Here are some common pediatric illnesses:

Infectious Diseases:

1. **Upper Respiratory Infections (URIs):**
   - **Common Agents:** Viruses like rhinovirus, and adenovirus.
   - **Symptoms:** Runny nose, cough, sore throat.
2. **Ear Infections (Otitis Media):**
   - **Common Agents:** Bacterial or viral infections.
   - **Symptoms:** Ear pain, fever, irritability.
3. **Strep Throat (Streptococcal Pharyngitis):**
   - **Common Agent:** Streptococcus bacteria.
   - **Symptoms:** Sore throat, fever, headache.
4. **Gastroenteritis:**
   - **Common Agents:** Viruses (rotavirus, norovirus) or bacteria.
   - **Symptoms:** Diarrhea, vomiting, abdominal pain.
5. **Urinary Tract Infections (UTIs):**
   - **Common Agents:** Bacterial infection, often E. coli.
   - **Symptoms:** Painful urination, frequent urination, fever.
6. **Chickenpox (Varicella):**
   - **Common Agent:** Varicella-zoster virus.
   - **Symptoms:** Itchy rash, fever, fatigue.
7. **Influenza (Flu):**
   - **Common Agent:** Influenza virus.

- ◦ **Symptoms:** Fever, body aches, respiratory symptoms.

8. **Hand, Foot, and Mouth Disease:**
   - ◦ **Common Agent:** Coxsackievirus.
   - ◦ **Symptoms:** Sores in the mouth, rash on hands and feet.

Chronic Conditions:

1. **Asthma:**
   - ◦ **Characteristics:** Chronic inflammation of the airways.
   - ◦ **Symptoms:** Wheezing, coughing, shortness of breath.

2. **Type 1 Diabetes:**
   - ◦ **Characteristics:** Autoimmune destruction of insulin-producing cells.
   - ◦ **Symptoms:** Excessive thirst, frequent urination, weight loss.

3. **Cystic Fibrosis:**
   - ◦ **Characteristics:** Genetic disorders affecting the respiratory and digestive systems.
   - ◦ **Symptoms:** Persistent cough, respiratory infections, digestive issues.

4. **Attention-Deficit/Hyperactivity Disorder (ADHD):**
   - ◦ **Characteristics:** Neurodevelopmental disorder affecting attention and impulse control.
   - ◦ **Symptoms:** Inattention, hyperactivity, impulsivity.

5. **Autism Spectrum Disorder (ASD):**
   - ◦ **Characteristics:** Neurodevelopmental disorder affecting social communication and behavior.

- ◦ **Symptoms:** Social challenges, repetitive behaviors, communication difficulties.

Acute Illnesses:

1. **Febrile Seizures:**
   - ◦ **Characteristics:** Seizures triggered by a sudden fever.
   - ◦ **Symptoms:** Convulsions, loss of consciousness during fever.
2. **Bronchiolitis:**
   - ◦ **Characteristics:** Inflammation of the small airways in the lungs.
   - ◦ **Symptoms:** Cough, wheezing, difficulty breathing.
3. **Gastroesophageal Reflux Disease (GERD):**
   - ◦ **Characteristics:** Chronic digestive disorder causing stomach acid to flow back into the esophagus.
   - ◦ **Symptoms:** Regurgitation, heartburn, irritability.
4. **Kawasaki Disease:**
   - ◦ **Characteristics:** Inflammation of blood vessels.
   - ◦ **Symptoms:** High fever, rash, swollen hands and feet.
5. **Pneumonia:**
   - ◦ **Characteristics:** Infection of the lungs.
   - ◦ **Symptoms:** Cough, fever, difficulty breathing.
6. **Meningitis:**
   - ◦ **Characteristics:** Inflammation of the membranes surrounding the brain and spinal cord.
   - ◦ **Symptoms:** Severe headache, fever, stiff neck.
7. **Acute Gastroenteritis:**
   - ◦ **Characteristics:** Sudden onset of gastrointestinal

inflammation.

◦ **Symptoms:** Diarrhea, vomiting, abdominal pain.

It's important to note that this list is not exhaustive, and each child may present with unique health challenges. Additionally, the management of pediatric illnesses often requires a collaborative approach involving pediatricians, pediatric nurses, and other healthcare professionals. Early detection, timely intervention, and appropriate management are crucial for ensuring the well-being of children with these conditions.

Pediatric Cancers

Pediatric cancers are a group of diseases characterized by the uncontrolled growth of abnormal cells in children. While cancer is relatively rare in children compared to adults, it remains a significant health concern. Pediatric cancers can occur in various parts of the body, and their types and treatments may differ from those seen in adults. Here are some common types of pediatric cancers:

1. Leukemia:

- **Common Types:** Acute lymphoblastic leukemia (ALL), acute myeloid leukemia (AML).
- **Characteristics:** Abnormal white blood cells multiply rapidly.
- **Symptoms:** Fatigue, fever, frequent infections, bruising, bone pain.

2. Brain and Central Nervous System (CNS) Tumors:

- **Common Types:** Medulloblastoma, gliomas, ependymomas.
- **Characteristics:** Tumors in the brain or spinal cord.
- **Symptoms:** Headaches, seizures, changes in behavior or coordination.

3. Neuroblastoma:

- **Characteristics:** Cancer forms in nerve tissue, usually in the adrenal glands.
- **Symptoms:** Abdominal pain, changes in bowel habits, weight loss.

4. Wilms Tumor:

- **Characteristics:** Kidney cancer that primarily affects children.
- **Symptoms:** Abdominal swelling or pain, fever.

5. Hepatoblastoma:

- **Characteristics:** Liver cancer in children.
- **Symptoms:** Abdominal mass, pain, jaundice.

6. Retinoblastoma:

- **Characteristics:** Eye cancer that affects the retina.
- **Symptoms:** White pupil (cat's eye reflex), crossed eyes, vision problems.

7. Osteosarcoma:

- **Characteristics:** Bone cancer, often occurring in the long bones.
- **Symptoms:** Bone pain, swelling, fractures.

8. Ewing Sarcoma:

- **Characteristics:** Rare bone cancer affecting the bones and surrounding tissues.
- **Symptoms:** Pain, swelling, fever.

9. Hodgkin Lymphoma:

- **Characteristics:** Cancer of the lymphatic system.
- **Symptoms:** Swollen lymph nodes, fatigue, fever, weight loss.

10. Non-Hodgkin Lymphoma:

- **Characteristics:** Cancer that originates in the lymphatic system but is not Hodgkin lymphoma.
- **Symptoms:** Swollen lymph nodes, abdominal pain, fever.

11. Rhabdomyosarcoma:

- **Characteristics:** Soft tissue cancer that forms in muscle tissue.
- **Symptoms:** Swelling or lump, pain, trouble urinating, or having bowel movements.

12. Germ Cell Tumors:

- **Common Types:** Teratomas, yolk sac tumors.
- **Characteristics:** Tumors that form from germ cells.
- **Symptoms:** Varies based on the location of the tumor.

13. Langerhans Cell Histiocytosis (LCH):

- **Characteristics:** Overproduction of Langerhans cells.
- **Symptoms:** Skin rash, bone lesions, swollen lymph nodes.

Treatment for pediatric cancers often involves a combination of surgery, chemotherapy, radiation therapy, immunotherapy, and targeted therapy. The specific approach depends on the type and stage of the cancer, as well as the child's overall health.

Pediatric oncology requires a multidisciplinary approach involving pediatric oncologists, surgeons, nurses, and other healthcare professionals. Advances in research and treatment have improved outcomes for many pediatric cancers, but ongoing research is essential to further enhance therapies and reduce long-term side effects.

Chapter 4

Childhood Immunizations

Childhood immunizations, also known as vaccinations or immunization schedules, are a crucial aspect of pediatric healthcare. Immunizations protect children from serious and potentially life-threatening diseases by stimulating the immune system to produce an immune response without causing the disease itself. The vaccination schedule is designed to provide optimal protection during a child's early years. Below are some common childhood immunizations:

1. Hepatitis B (HepB):

- **Recommended Doses:** Birth, 1-2 months, 6-18 months.
- **Disease:** Hepatitis B, a viral infection affecting the liver.

2. Rotavirus (RV):

- **Recommended Doses:** 2 months, 4 months, 6 months.
- **Disease:** Severe diarrhea and vomiting caused by the rotavirus.

3. Diphtheria, Tetanus, and Pertussis (DTaP):

- **Recommended Doses:** 2 months, 4 months, 6 months, 15-18 months, 4-6 years.
- **Diseases:** Diphtheria, tetanus, and whooping cough (pertussis).

4. Haemophilus Influenzae Type b (Hib):

- **Recommended Doses:** 2 months, 4 months, 6 months, 12-15 months.
- **Disease:** Invasive disease caused by Haemophilus influenzae type b.

5. Pneumococcal Conjugate (PCV13):

- **Recommended Doses:** 2 months, 4 months, 6 months, 12-15 months.
- **Diseases:** Infections caused by Streptococcus pneumoniae.

6. Polio (IPV):

- **Recommended Doses:** 2 months, 4 months, 6-18 months, 4-6 years.

- **Disease:** Polio, a viral illness affecting the nervous system.

7. Influenza (Flu):

- **Recommended Doses:** Annually starting at 6 months.
- **Disease:** Seasonal influenza caused by influenza viruses.

8. Measles, Mumps, and Rubella (MMR):

- **Recommended Doses:** 1st dose at 12-15 months, 2nd dose at 4-6 years.
- **Diseases:** Measles, mumps, and rubella.

9. Varicella (VAR):

- **Recommended Doses:** 1st dose at 12-15 months, 2nd dose at 4-6 years.
- **Disease:** Chickenpox, a highly contagious viral infection.

Parents and caregivers need to follow the recommended immunization schedule provided by healthcare professionals. Vaccines protect not only the individual but also contribute to community immunity, preventing the spread of diseases within populations. Regular check-ups with pediatricians or healthcare providers help ensure that children receive the appropriate vaccinations at the right time.

Understanding and Administering Vaccines

Understanding and administering vaccines is a critical aspect of healthcare, as vaccines play a key role in preventing and controlling infectious diseases. Here are the key components of understanding and administering vaccines:

Understanding Vaccines:

1. **Vaccine Basics:**
   - **Definition:** Vaccines are biological products that stimulate the immune system to produce an immune response, protecting against specific diseases.
   - **Components:** Vaccines may contain weakened or inactivated pathogens, pieces of pathogens, or synthetic components that mimic pathogens.

2. **Types of Vaccines:**
   - **Live Attenuated Vaccines:** Weakened forms of the virus or bacteria (e.g., measles, mumps, rubella).
   - **Inactivated Vaccines:** Pathogens that have been killed (e.g., polio, hepatitis A).
   - **Subunit, Recombinant, or Conjugate Vaccines:** Contain specific pieces of the pathogen (e.g., Hepatitis B, Haemophilus influenzae type b).
   - **mRNA Vaccines:** Contain a small piece of the pathogen's genetic material to stimulate an immune response (e.g., COVID-19 vaccines).

3. **Vaccine Immunology:**
   - **Primary Goal:** Induce an immune response without causing the disease.

- **Memory Cells:** Create immunological memory for long-term protection.

4. **Herd Immunity:**
   - **Definition:** When a high percentage of a population is immune to a disease, it provides indirect protection to those who are not immune.
   - **Achieving Herd Immunity:** Typically, through widespread vaccination.

Administering Vaccines:

1. **Vaccine Storage and Handling:**
   - **Cold Chain:** Maintain the recommended temperature range during storage and transportation to preserve vaccine potency.
   - **Vaccine Refrigerators:** Regular monitoring, temperature logs, and backup plans in case of power failure.

2. **Vaccine Administration Techniques:**
   - **Intramuscular (IM) Injection:** Common for many vaccines, typically administered into the deltoid muscle.
   - **Subcutaneous (SC) Injection:** Used for some vaccines, injected into the fatty layer just beneath the skin.
   - **Intradermal (ID) Injection:** Injected into the dermis layer of the skin; less common.

3. **Injection Site and Needle Selection:**
   - **Deltoid Muscle:** Preferred site for most vaccines in adults.
   - **Thigh:** Common site for infants and young

children.

- **Needle Length:** Varied based on age, muscle mass, and route of administration.

4. **Preparation and Reconstitution:**
   - **Single-dose vials:** Ready for use.
   - **Multidose Vials:** This may require reconstitution (mixing) before administration.

5. **Patient Education and Consent:**
   - **Informed Consent:** Explain the benefits and risks of the vaccine to the patient or parent/guardian.
   - **Addressing Concerns:** Provide accurate information about vaccine safety and efficacy.

6. **Documentation and Reporting:**
   - **Vaccine Records:** Maintain accurate records of administered vaccines.
   - **Vaccine Information Statements (VIS):** Provide relevant information to patients before vaccination.
   - **Adverse Events Reporting:** Report any adverse events following vaccination to the appropriate authorities.

7. **Post-Vaccination Observation:**
   - **Observation Period:** Monitor individuals for a brief period after vaccination to detect any immediate adverse reactions.
   - **Guidelines:** Follow recommended observation periods based on the type of vaccine.

8. **Follow-Up Vaccinations:**
   - **Booster Doses:** Some vaccines require booster doses for continued immunity.
   - **Catch-Up Vaccination:** For individuals who missed

scheduled vaccinations.

Understanding and administering vaccines require adherence to established protocols, maintaining proper storage conditions, and effective communication with patients or their caregivers. Healthcare providers should stay informed about updated vaccine recommendations and guidelines to ensure the safe and effective administration of vaccines.

Immunization Schedules

Immunization schedules provide a timeline for when children and adults should receive specific vaccines. These schedules are developed by public health authorities and medical organizations to ensure optimal protection against infectious diseases. It's important to note that vaccine schedules may vary slightly based on the country and region. Below are general guidelines for immunization schedules for children and adults in the United States:

Childhood Immunization Schedule (United States):

Birth to 6 Years:

1. **Hepatitis B (HepB):**
   - Birth
   - 1-2 months
   - 6-18 months
2. **Rotavirus (RV):**
   - 2 months
   - 4 months
   - 6 months
3. **Diphtheria, Tetanus, and Pertussis (DTaP):**
   - 2 months
   - 4 months
   - 6 months
   - 15-18 months
   - 4-6 years
4. **Haemophilus Influenzae Type b (Hib):**
   - 2 months
   - 4 months
   - 6 months
   - 12-15 months
5. **Pneumococcal Conjugate (PCV13):**

- 2 months
- 4 months
- 6 months
- 12-15 months

6. **Inactivated Poliovirus (IPV):**
   - 2 months
   - 4 months
   - 6-18 months
   - 4-6 years

7. **Influenza (Flu):**
   - Annually starting at 6 months

8. **Measles, Mumps, Rubella (MMR):**
   - 1st dose at 12-15 months
   - 2nd dose at 4-6 years

9. **Varicella (VAR):**
   - 1st dose at 12-15 months
   - 2nd dose at 4-6 years

10. **Hepatitis A (HepA):**
    - 1st dose at 12-23 months
    - 2nd dose 6-18 months later

7 to 18 Years:

1. **Tetanus, Diphtheria, Pertussis (Tdap):**
   - 11-12 years (boost every 10 years)

2. **Meningococcal (MenACWY):**
   - 11-12 years
   - Booster at 16 years

3. **Human Papillomavirus (HPV):**
   - Series starting at 11-12 years (two or three doses, depending on age at first dose)

4. **Influenza (Flu):**
   - Annually

Adult Immunization Schedule (United States):

1. **Influenza (Flu):**
   - Annually
2. **Tetanus, Diphtheria, Pertussis (Tdap):**
   - One-time Tdap, followed by Td booster every 10 years
3. **Human Papillomavirus (HPV):**
   - Up to age 26 for males and females
4. **Pneumococcal (Pneumonia):**
   - For adults 65 and older or those with certain health conditions
5. **Shingles (Herpes Zoster):**
   - For adults 50 and older
6. **Hepatitis B (HepB):**
   - For adults at risk due to occupation, lifestyle, or health conditions
7. **Hepatitis A (HepA):**
   - For adults at risk due to occupation, lifestyle, or health conditions
8. **Measles, Mumps, Rubella (MMR):**
   - If born after 1957 and not previously vaccinated
9. **Meningococcal:**
   - For certain high-risk individuals
10. **Varicella (Chickenpox):**
    - For adults without evidence of immunity

It's essential to consult with healthcare providers to ensure that individuals receive the appropriate vaccinations based on their health status, age, and potential exposure risks. Immunization schedules may be updated periodically to reflect advances in vaccine research and changing epidemiological patterns.

Chapter 5

Pediatric Pharmacology

Pediatric pharmacology refers to the study of how drugs interact with the bodies of infants, children, and adolescents. It is a specialized branch of pharmacology that focuses on the unique aspects of drug administration, pharmacokinetics (how drugs move through the body), and pharmacodynamics (how drugs exert their effects) in the pediatric population. Children are not simply small adults, and their developing bodies have distinct characteristics that impact drug responses. Here are some key considerations in pediatric pharmacology:

1. Age-Related Changes:

- **Neonates and Infants:** Limited hepatic and renal function; immature blood-brain barrier.
- **Young Children:** Continued maturation of organ systems.
- **Adolescents:** Approach adult physiological function.

2. Dosage Considerations:

- **Weight-Based Dosing:** Many medications are dosed according to the child's weight.
- **Body Surface Area (BSA):** Some chemotherapy drugs and specific medications are dosed based on BSA.

3. Oral Medications:

- **Liquid Formulations:** Often preferred due to ease of dose adjustment.
- **Flavoring Agents:** Used to enhance palatability.

4. Intravenous (IV) Medications:

- **Vascular Access:** Considerations for the type of vascular access, especially in infants.
- **Infusion Rates:** Based on age and weight.

5. Pharmacokinetic Differences:

- **Absorption:** Gastric pH, gastric emptying time, and intestinal transit time vary in children.
- **Distribution:** Changes in body composition (lean body mass and fat), protein binding, and organ

perfusion.

- **Metabolism:** Enzyme systems in the liver may be immature, leading to slower drug metabolism.
- **Elimination:** Renal function is less efficient in neonates and infants, impacting drug clearance.

6. Safety Considerations:

- **Drug Formulations:** Avoid formulations with high alcohol content or other potentially harmful additives.
- **Allergies and Adverse Reactions:** Monitor for allergic reactions or adverse effects, as children may have difficulty expressing symptoms.

7. Pediatric Formularies:

- **Specialized Drug Formularies:** Developed to guide appropriate medication use in pediatrics.
- **Pediatric Dosage Handbook:** Resource for dosing information.

8. Neonatal Pharmacology:

- **Neonatal Intensive Care Units (NICUs):** Specialized considerations for premature infants with unique pharmacokinetic and pharmacodynamic characteristics.
- **Medication Safety:** Dilution and concentration calculations are critical.

9. Behavioral and Psychosocial Considerations:

- **Child-Friendly Formulations:** Flavored medications, chewable tablets, or oral disintegrating tablets.
- **Dosing Challenges:** Children may resist medication administration.

10. Antibiotic Stewardship:

- **Appropriate Use:** Consideration of microbial resistance and potential long-term effects on the microbiome.
- **Dosage Adjustments:** Ensuring therapeutic levels are achieved.

11. Educating Parents and Caregivers:

- **Medication Administration:** Instructing parents on proper administration techniques.
- **Monitoring for Adverse Effects:** Providing information on signs and symptoms to watch for.

12. Research and Development:

- **Ethical Considerations:** Conducting pediatric clinical trials with attention to ethical principles.

- **Age-Appropriate Formulations:** Ongoing research to develop medications suitable for children.

Pediatric pharmacology requires a nuanced and individualized approach, considering the child's age, weight, organ maturity, and specific health conditions. Collaboration between healthcare providers, pharmacists, and parents is crucial to ensure safe and effective medication management in the pediatric population. Additionally, ongoing research in this field contributes to improved drug safety and efficacy for children.

Medication Administration for Children

Administering medications to children requires careful consideration of the child's age, weight, developmental stage, and the specific characteristics of the medication. Here are some general guidelines for medication administration in children:

1. Dosage Calculation:

- **Weight-Based Dosing:** Calculate medication doses based on the child's weight.
- **Body Surface Area (BSA):** Some medications, especially chemotherapy drugs, may be dosed based on BSA.

2. Formulation Considerations:

- **Liquid Formulations:** Preferred for infants and young children who may have difficulty swallowing pills.
- **Chewable Tablets or Disintegrating Tablets:** Appropriate for older children who can chew or let the tablet dissolve.

3. Oral Medication Administration:

- **Use an Appropriate Syringe or Dropper:** Ensure accurate measurement for liquid medications.
- **Avoid Household Spoons:** Use calibrated measuring devices provided with the medication.

4. Flavoring Agents:

- **Flavored Medications:** Some pharmacies offer flavored options to improve palatability.
- **Consider Preferences:** Ask the child or parent about flavor preferences when available.

5. Intravenous (IV) Medication Administration:

- **Vascular Access:** Consider the type of vascular access, especially in infants.
- **Infusion Rates:** Adjust based on the child's age and weight.

6. Injection Sites:

- **Intramuscular (IM) Injections:** Commonly used in older children; choose an appropriate muscle (e.g., deltoid or thigh).

- **Subcutaneous (SC) Injections:** Used for certain medications; typically administered in the fatty layer just beneath the skin.

7. Topical Medication Application:

- **Skin Preparation:** Ensure the skin is clean and dry before applying topical medications.
- **Avoid Broken Skin:** Do not apply medications to broken or irritated skin unless directed.

8. Eye and Ear Drops:

- **Eye Drops:** Aim for the conjunctival sac; avoid touching the dropper to the eye.
- **Ear Drops:** Administer in the ear canal; straighten the ear canal in young children by pulling the earlobe backward and downward.

9. Nasal Sprays:

- **Positioning:** Ensure the child's head is in an upright position.
- **Proper Technique:** Instruct the child to breathe in slowly through the nose while administering the spray.

10. Behavioral and Psychosocial Considerations:

- **Distraction Techniques:** Engage the child in a favorite activity or use toys to distract them during administration.
- **Use Positive Reinforcement:** Praise the child for cooperation.

11. Medication Safety:

- **Check Allergies:** Confirm the child's allergies before administering any medication.
- **Double-check dosages:** Confirm the correct dosage with another healthcare professional if there are any doubts.

12. Educate Parents and Caregivers:

- **Clear Instructions:** Provide clear instructions on how to administer medications at home.
- **Ask About Preferences:** Inquire about any challenges or preferences related to medication administration.

13. Recordkeeping:

- **Maintain Accurate Records:** Document the date, time, and dosage of each administered medication.
- **Communication:** Ensure communication with parents and healthcare providers regarding medication administration.

14. Adverse Effects Monitoring:

- **Educate Caregivers:** Inform parents and caregivers about potential side effects to monitor.
- **Seek Medical Attention:** Advise caregivers on when to seek medical attention for adverse reactions.

15. Safety with Liquid Medications:

- **Use a Medication Syringe:** For accurate measurement, especially for small doses.
- **Avoid Mixing with Food:** Unless approved by the healthcare provider.

16. Child-Friendly Approach:

- **Use Age-Appropriate Language:** Explain procedures in a way that the child can understand.
- **Involve the Child:** Depending on age, involve the child in the process and encourage independence.

17. Patient and Family Education:

- **Medication Understanding:** Ensure parents and caregivers understand the purpose, dose, and potential side effects of the medication.
- **Written Instructions:** Provide written instructions for home administration.

18. Consideration of Cultural and Ethical Factors:

- **Cultural Competence:** Understand and respect cultural preferences related to medication administration.
- **Ethical Considerations:** Ensure informed consent and respect the child's autonomy as appropriate.

19. Intranasal Medication Administration:

- **Proper Technique:** Administer intranasal medications with proper technique, especially in young children.

20. Collaboration with the Child:

- **Assess Child's Understanding:** Depending on age, assess the child's understanding and willingness to participate in their care.

- **Address Fears or Concerns:** Acknowledge and address any fears or concerns the child may have.

21. Emergency Preparedness:

- **Knowledge of Emergency Measures:** Healthcare providers and caregivers should be aware of emergency measures in case of accidental ingestion or adverse reactions.

Note:

Always follow the healthcare provider's orders and medication administration guidelines. Dosages, routes of administration, and considerations may vary based on the specific medication, the child's health status, and the healthcare provider's instructions. Pediatric medication administration requires a patient-centered and family-centered approach, considering the child's developmental stage and individual needs.

Dosage Calculations and Considerations

Dosage calculations are a crucial aspect of medication administration, ensuring that patients receive the correct amount of medication based on their characteristics. Here are key considerations and methods for dosage calculations:

1. Dosage Calculation Methods:

a. Body Weight-Based Dosage:

- Many medications are dosed based on the patient's weight.
- Common formulas include mg/kg (milligrams per kilogram) or mcg/kg (micrograms per kilogram).

Example:

- If the prescribed dose is 10 mg/kg, and the child's weight is 20 kg:
  - ◇◇◇◇=10 mg/kg×20 kg=200 mg$Dose$=10mg/kg×20kg=200mg

b. Body Surface Area (BSA)-Based Dosage:

- Some medications, especially in oncology, are dosed based on BSA.
- The Mosteller formula is commonly used: (height in cm×weight in kg3600) (3600height in cm×weight in kg).

Example:

- If BSA is calculated as 1.5 m^2 and the prescribed dose is 100 mg/m^2:
  - ◇◇◇◇=100 mg/m2×1.5 m2=150 mg$Dose$=100mg/m2×1.5m2=150mg

c. Volume-Based Dosage:

- Liquid medications are often dosed based on volume (e.g., ml or cc).
- Use concentration (mg/ml) to calculate the volume.

Example:

- If the prescribed dose is 50 mg, and the concentration is 10 mg/ml:

  - $\blacklozenge\blacklozenge\blacklozenge\blacklozenge\blacklozenge\blacklozenge$ =DoseConcentration=50 mg10 mg/ml=5 ml$Volume$=ConcentrationDose=10mg/ml50mg=5ml

2. Considerations for Dosage Calculations:
a. Medication Formulation:

- **Solid Dosage Forms:** Tablets, capsules.
- **Liquid Dosage Forms:** Solutions, suspensions.

b. Concentration:

- **Medication Strength:** Check the concentration of the medication (e.g., mg/ml).
- **Conversion if Necessary:** Convert concentrations to match the prescribed dose unit.

c. Patient Characteristics:

- **Age:** Consider age-related differences in drug metabolism.
- **Renal and Hepatic Function:** Adjust dosage for impaired renal or hepatic function.

d. Prescription Orders:

- **Review Orders:** Carefully review the prescription for accuracy.
- **Units of Measurement:** Ensure consistency in units (e.g., mg, mcg).

e. Unit Conversion:

- **Convert Units if Needed:** Ensure that all units are consistent for calculations.

f. Safety Margins:

- **Check Maximum Doses:** Be aware of the maximum recommended doses to avoid toxicity.
- **Consider Safety Margins:** Factor in safety margins for pediatric patients.

g. Route of Administration:

- **Oral, Intravenous, Intramuscular, etc.:** Different routes may require different dosage calculations.

h. Infusion Rates:

- **Intravenous Infusions:** Calculate infusion rates based on the desired dose and duration.

i. Drug Interactions:

- **Check for Interactions:** Be aware of potential drug interactions that may affect dosage requirements.

j. Pediatric Considerations:

- **Dosage Adjustments for Pediatrics:** Children may require weight-based or age-specific adjustments.
- **Liquid Formulations:** Preferred for accurate dosing in pediatric patients.

k. Geriatric Considerations:

- **Altered Pharmacokinetics:** Consider changes in drug metabolism and elimination in elderly patients.

3. Practical Examples:
a. Weight-Based Dosage:

- If the prescribed dose is 0.2 mg/kg, and the patient weighs 70 kg:
  - ◆◆◆◆=0.2 mg/kg×70 kg=14 mg$Dose$=0.2mg/kg×70kg=14mg

b. Volume-Based Dosage:

- If the prescribed dose is 25 mg, and the concentration is 5 mg/ml:
  - ◆◆◆◆◆◆=DoseConcentration=25 mg5 mg/ml=5 ml$Volume$=ConcentrationDose =5mg/ml25mg=5ml

4. Electronic Calculators:

- Utilize electronic calculators or pharmacy software to minimize the risk of calculation errors.

Dosage calculations require attention to detail, adherence to proper measurement units, and consideration of patient-specific factors. Healthcare providers should always follow established protocols, use reliable resources, and double-check calculations to ensure patient safety. Additionally, consultation with a pharmacist or other healthcare professionals can guide dosage calculations and considerations.

Chapter 6

Family-Centered Care

Family-centered care is an approach to healthcare that recognizes the importance of involving patients and their families as active participants in the healthcare process. This model of care emphasizes collaboration, communication, and partnership between healthcare providers, patients, and their families to ensure the best possible outcomes. Family-centered care is particularly relevant in pediatric healthcare but can be applied across various healthcare settings. Here are the key principles and components of family-centered care:

1. Respect for the Family as a Unit:

- Recognize the family as a fundamental unit of care.
- Understand and acknowledge the diversity of family structures.

2. Collaborative Partnerships:

- Establish collaborative partnerships between healthcare providers and families.
- Encourage shared decision-making and mutual respect.

3. Information Sharing and Communication:

- Foster open and transparent communication between healthcare providers and families.
- Share information in a way that is easily understandable to the family.

4. Inclusion of Family Perspectives:

- Seek and incorporate the perspectives, preferences, and values of the family in the care plan.
- Encourage families to actively participate in discussions about care goals and treatment plans.

5. Individualized and Culturally Competent Care:

- Provide care that is tailored to the individual needs of each family.
- Be sensitive to cultural, religious, and linguistic diversity.

6. Support for Family Strengths:

- Recognize and build upon the strengths and resilience of the family.
- Empower families to be active participants in the care of their loved ones.

7. Continuous and Coordinated Care:

- Ensure continuity of care by involving families in care transitions and discharge planning.
- Coordinate care across different healthcare providers and settings.

8. Emotional and Psychosocial Support:

- Address the emotional and psychosocial needs of both the patient and the family.
- Provide resources and support for coping with the challenges of illness.

9. Family Presence and Participation:

- Encourage family presence during medical rounds, consultations, and procedures when appropriate.
- Support family participation in caregiving activities.

10. Shared Care Planning:

- Collaborate with families to develop care plans that align with their goals and priorities.
- Include families in the decision-making process regarding

treatment options.

11. Advocacy for Family Needs:

- Advocate for the needs and preferences of the family within the healthcare system.
- Empower families to advocate for their loved ones.

12. Education and Support:

- Provide clear and comprehensive education to families about the patient's condition and treatment plan.
- Offer ongoing support and resources for learning about the healthcare process.

13. Flexible and Responsive Care:

- Be flexible and responsive to the changing needs of the family and the patient.
- Adjust care plans based on feedback and evolving circumstances.

14. Respect for Privacy and Dignity:

- Respect the privacy and dignity of the family, recognizing that they are integral to the care team.
- Establish trust and rapport with families to create a supportive environment.

15. Evaluation and Feedback:

- Seek feedback from families about their experiences with care.
- Use evaluations to continuously improve the quality of family-centered care.

Family-centered care is an inclusive and collaborative approach that recognizes the interconnectedness of individuals within a family unit. It promotes a holistic understanding of healthcare, taking into account not only the medical needs of the patient but also the social, emotional, and cultural aspects of their lives. This model of care has been associated with improved patient and family satisfaction, better adherence to treatment plans, and positive health outcomes.

Involving and Educating Families in the Care Process

Involving and educating families in the care process is essential for providing comprehensive and effective healthcare, particularly in pediatric settings. When families are active participants in the care of their loved ones, it can lead to better outcomes, increased satisfaction, and improved adherence to treatment plans. Here are strategies for involving and educating families in the care process:

Involvement of Families:

1. **Family-Centered Rounds:**
   - Include families in bedside rounds to discuss the patient's condition, treatment plan, and goals.
   - Encourage questions and address concerns during these rounds.
2. **Shared Decision-Making:**
   - Involve families in decisions about the care plan, treatment options, and discharge planning.
   - Provide information about potential risks and benefits to facilitate informed decision-making.
3. **Care Planning Meetings:**
   - Schedule family meetings to discuss the overall care plan, including goals, milestones, and expected outcomes.
   - Collaborate with families to set realistic expectations and address their priorities.
4. **Patient and Family Advisory Councils:**
   - Establish advisory councils comprised of patients and family members to provide feedback on healthcare policies, procedures, and services.
   - Include families in the development of patient

education materials.

5. **Encouraging Presence:**
   - Facilitate family presence during medical procedures, treatments, and consultations when appropriate.
   - Encourage family members to actively participate in caregiving activities.

6. **Family Support Groups:**
   - Connect families with support groups where they can share experiences and insights.
   - Support groups can provide emotional support and practical advice.

7. **Care Conferences:**
   - Conduct care conferences with the involvement of healthcare providers, families, and other relevant stakeholders.
   - Use these conferences to discuss complex cases and address multidisciplinary aspects of care.

8. **Cultural Competency:**
   - Be aware of and respect the cultural, religious, and linguistic diversity of families.
   - Consider cultural preferences when developing care plans.

Education for Families:

1. **Clear and Accessible Communication:**
   - Use plain language to explain medical information and treatment plans.
   - Provide written materials and educational resources in a language and format that is accessible to the family.

2. **Teaching Sessions:**

- Conduct individualized teaching sessions for families to explain specific aspects of care, such as medication administration or wound care.
- Encourage questions and ensure understanding before discharge.

3. **Electronic Health Records Access:**
   - Provide families with access to electronic health records when possible.
   - Enable families to review test results, treatment plans, and other relevant information.

4. **Home Care Instructions:**
   - Offer detailed instructions for care at home, including medication administration, signs of complications, and follow-up appointments.
   - Provide a written care plan for reference.

5. **Online Resources:**
   - Direct families to reputable online resources for additional information and support.
   - Share educational websites or videos related to the patient's condition.

6. **Peer Support:**
   - Connect families with peers who have experienced similar healthcare journeys.
   - Peer support can provide valuable insights and practical advice.

7. **Simulation and Practice:**
   - Use simulation or hands-on practice to teach families certain healthcare procedures.
   - Ensure families feel confident and capable of providing care at home.

8. **Post-Discharge Follow-Up:**
   - Schedule post-discharge follow-up appointments to

assess the patient's progress and address any concerns.

- ○ Reinforce important aspects of care during follow-up visits.

9. **24/7 Helplines:**
- ○ Provide access to a 24/7 helpline or on-call service for families to seek guidance or ask questions.
- ○ Offer a reliable point of contact for urgent concerns.

10. **Interactive Materials:**
- ○ Use interactive materials, such as diagrams or models, to visually explain medical concepts.
- ○ Tailor educational materials to the specific learning preferences of the family.

Evaluation and Continuous Improvement:

1. **Feedback Mechanisms:**
- ○ Establish feedback mechanisms to gather input from families about their experiences with care and education.
- ○ Use surveys, interviews, or focus groups to collect feedback.

2. **Quality Improvement Initiatives:**
- ○ Use feedback and data to drive quality improvement initiatives.
- ○ Address identified areas for improvement in family involvement and education.

3. **Regular Training for Healthcare Providers:**
- ○ Provide ongoing training for healthcare providers on effective communication and collaboration with families.
- ○ Encourage a culture of continuous learning.

4. **Celebrate Successes:**

- ◦ Acknowledge and celebrate successes in family involvement and education.
- ◦ Share success stories to inspire and motivate both healthcare providers and families.

Involving and educating families in the care process is a collaborative effort that requires effective communication, cultural sensitivity, and a commitment to partnership between healthcare providers and families. By recognizing families as essential members of the care team, healthcare organizations can enhance the overall quality of care and promote positive outcomes for patients.

Communication Strategies with Parents and Guardians

Effective communication with parents and guardians is crucial in healthcare, particularly in pediatric settings. Clear and open communication builds trust, promotes collaboration, and ensures that families are actively engaged in the care process. Here are communication strategies that healthcare providers can employ when interacting with parents and guardians:

1. Active Listening:

- **Demonstrate Engagement:** Give full attention, make eye contact, and show that you are actively listening.
- **Use Verbal and Nonverbal Cues:** Nodding, paraphrasing, and providing feedback demonstrate active listening.

2. Empathy and Compassion:

- **Acknowledge Emotions:** Recognize and validate the emotions of parents and guardians.
- **Express Understanding:** Use empathetic statements to convey understanding and support.

3. Clear and Simple Language:

- **Avoid Medical Jargon:** Use layman's terms and avoid medical jargon to ensure understanding.
- **Check for Understanding:** Encourage questions and ask parents to summarize information to confirm comprehension.

4. Establishing Rapport:

- **Introduce Yourself:** Begin interactions by introducing yourself and your role.
- **Build Trust:** Establish trust through warmth, respect, and a non-judgmental attitude.

5. Cultural Competence:

- **Understand Cultural Differences:** Be aware of cultural nuances and tailor communication accordingly.
- **Ask About Preferences:** Inquire about communication preferences and the use of interpreters if

necessary.

6. Shared Decision-Making:

- **Involve Parents in Decisions:** Engage parents in shared decision-making regarding their child's care.
- **Provide Options:** Present treatment options and discuss pros and cons.

7. Regular Updates:

- **Timely Communication:** Provide regular updates on the child's condition and treatment plan.
- **Scheduled Meetings:** Schedule regular meetings to discuss progress and address concerns.

8. Use of Visual Aids:

- **Diagrams and Charts:** Use visual aids to explain medical concepts or treatment procedures.
- **Show and Tell:** Physically demonstrate equipment or procedures when appropriate.

9. Written Information:

- **Provide Written Materials:** Offer written instructions, care plans, and educational materials.
- **Use Readable Fonts:** Ensure that written materials use clear and readable fonts.

10. Encourage Questions:

- **Open Door Policy:** Encourage parents to ask questions and express concerns.
- **Ask for Questions:** Promptly ask if there are any questions after providing information.

11. Consistent Team Communication:

- **Care Coordination:** Ensure consistent communication among the healthcare team.
- **Unified Messages:** Present a unified message to parents to avoid confusion.

12. Respect Privacy:

- **Private Conversations:** Hold sensitive discussions in private settings.
- **Ask About Preferences:** Inquire about the level of privacy parents prefer during discussions.

13. Addressing Concerns:

- **Be Open to Feedback:** Create an environment where parents feel comfortable providing feedback.

- **Promptly Address Concerns:** Address any concerns or issues promptly.

14. Collaborative Goal-Setting:

- **Establish Common Goals:** Work collaboratively with parents to set common goals for the child's care.
- **Acknowledge Parental Expertise:** Recognize and respect the expertise parents bring to their child's care.

15. Use of Technology:

- **Virtual Communication:** Utilize virtual communication methods for updates or discussions when needed.
- **Secure Communication:** Ensure that any electronic communication complies with privacy regulations.

16. Post-Visit Summaries:

- **Summarize Discussions:** Provide a summary of discussions and next steps at the end of visits.
- **Written Follow-Up:** Send a written summary or care plan after important discussions.

17. Acknowledging Time Constraints:

- **Set Expectations:** Be transparent about time constraints and set realistic expectations for discussions.
- **Offer Follow-Up:** Offer additional time or follow-up opportunities if needed.

18. Be Mindful of Nonverbal Cues:

- **Body Language:** Pay attention to your own and parents' body language.
- **Facial Expressions:** Be aware of facial expressions that may convey emotions.

19. Emergency Communication Plan:

- **Provide Emergency Contacts:** Ensure parents have emergency contact information and know how to reach healthcare providers in urgent situations.
- **Clarify Emergency Procedures:** Communicate emergency procedures and what actions parents should take.

20. Educational Workshops:

- **Offer Workshops:** Conduct workshops or informational sessions on relevant healthcare topics for parents.

- **Interactive Sessions:** Include interactive components to engage parents in learning.

Effective communication with parents and guardians is an ongoing process that requires adaptability, cultural sensitivity, and a commitment to collaboration. Tailoring communication to individual preferences and ensuring that parents feel informed and involved can contribute to a positive healthcare experience for both the family and the healthcare team.

Chapter 7

Pediatric Emergency Care

Pediatric emergency care involves the specialized medical attention and treatment provided to infants, children, and adolescents who require urgent medical intervention due to illness or injury. Providing emergency care to pediatric patients requires a unique set of skills, knowledge, and considerations due to the developmental differences and specific needs of children. Here are key aspects of pediatric emergency care:

1. Recognition of Pediatric Emergencies:

- **Knowledge of Pediatric Warning Signs:** Recognize signs of pediatric emergencies, including respiratory distress, altered mental status, severe dehydration, and signs of shock.
- **Age-Specific Considerations:** Understand age-specific variations in vital signs and symptoms.

2. Pediatric Assessment Triangle (PAT):

- **Appearance, Work of Breathing, and Circulation:** Use the PAT to rapidly assess the overall condition of a pediatric patient.
- **Quick Initial Assessment:** Provides a quick and structured approach to identifying critical conditions.

3. Airway Management:

- **Age-Appropriate Airway Techniques:** Use age-appropriate airway management techniques, considering anatomical and physiological differences.
- **Recognize Signs of Airway Obstruction:** Promptly identify and address signs of airway obstruction, such as stridor or respiratory distress.

4. Respiratory Distress and Failure:

- **Use of Pediatric Resuscitation Bag-Mask:** Utilize age-appropriate bag-mask ventilation for respiratory support.
- **Recognize Signs of Respiratory Failure:** Identify signs of respiratory distress and failure, such as retractions, nasal flaring, and grunting.

5. Vascular Access and Fluid Resuscitation:

75

- **Appropriate Intravenous (IV) Access:** Establish IV access for fluid administration or medication delivery.
- **Calculate Pediatric Fluid Resuscitation:** Calculate fluid resuscitation volumes based on weight and clinical condition.

6. Pain Management:

- **Age-Appropriate Pain Assessment:** Use age-specific pain assessment tools to evaluate pain.
- **Medication Dosing:** Administer pain medications at appropriate doses for pediatric patients.

7. Temperature Control:

- **Temperature Monitoring:** Regularly monitor and manage body temperature, especially in infants and young children.
- **Cooling Measures:** Implement cooling measures for patients with fever or hyperthermia.

8. Child Life Specialists:

- **Incorporate Child Life Specialists:** Utilize child life specialists to provide emotional support, distraction, and coping strategies for pediatric patients.
- **Reduce Anxiety:** Minimize stress and anxiety during emergency procedures through play therapy and other interventions.

9. Pediatric Equipment and Supplies:

- **Size-Appropriate Equipment:** Ensure availability of size-appropriate equipment, including airway devices, defibrillator pads, and monitoring tools.
- **Pediatric Drug Formulary:** Maintain a pediatric drug formulary for accurate medication administration.

10. Transport Considerations:

- **Pediatric Transport Teams:** Consider specialized pediatric transport teams for interfacility transfers.
- **Stabilization Before Transport:** Stabilize the patient before transport, addressing immediate life-threatening issues.

11. Family-Centered Care:

- **Family Presence:** Allow and encourage family presence during resuscitation efforts when appropriate.
- **Communication with Parents:** Communicate clearly and compassionately with parents, providing updates on the child's condition.

12. Neonatal Resuscitation:

- **Neonatal Resuscitation Program (NRP):** Healthcare providers should be trained in neonatal resuscitation techniques.
- **Umbilical Venous Access:** Consider umbilical venous access in neonatal emergencies.

13. Trauma Care:

- **Pediatric Trauma Assessment:** Conduct a thorough trauma assessment, recognizing common pediatric injuries.
- **Age-Specific Injury Patterns:** Be aware of age-specific injury patterns, such as abusive head trauma in infants.

14. Pediatric Advanced Life Support (PALS):

- **PALS Training:** Healthcare providers should be trained in PALS, which includes advanced life support interventions for pediatric emergencies.
- **Algorithm-Based Approach:** Use PALS algorithms to guide resuscitation efforts.

15. Ethical Considerations:

- **Family Consent:** Obtain informed consent from parents or legal guardians for medical procedures.
- **End-of-Life Care:** Engage in compassionate end-of-life care discussions when necessary.

16. Cultural Sensitivity:

- **Cultural Competence:** Demonstrate cultural competence in emergency care, respecting diverse beliefs and practices.
- **Interpreter Services:** Use interpreter services if language barriers exist.

17. Quality Improvement and Simulation:

- **Regular Drills and Simulation:** Conduct regular drills and simulation exercises to enhance the team's readiness for pediatric emergencies.

- **Review and Debrief:** After each pediatric emergency, conduct a thorough review and debriefing session to identify areas for improvement.

Pediatric emergency care requires a multidisciplinary and collaborative approach, involving healthcare providers, families, and support staff. Ongoing training, simulation exercises, and a commitment to continuous improvement are essential elements in providing optimal care to pediatric patients during emergencies.

Recognizing and Managing Pediatric Emergencies

Recognizing and managing pediatric emergencies requires a combination of clinical knowledge, rapid assessment skills, and effective communication. Pediatric patients have unique physiological and developmental considerations, making it crucial for healthcare providers to be well-prepared for various emergencies. Here are some key pediatric emergencies and general principles for recognition and management:

1. Respiratory Emergencies:

- Recognition:
  - Rapid breathing, grunting, retractions, nasal flaring.
  - Cyanosis or pallor.
  - Altered mental status.
- Management:
  - Maintain open airway.
  - Administer oxygen.
  - Consider nebulized medications.
  - Be prepared for possible intubation or advanced airway management.

2. Cardiac Arrest:

- Recognition:
  - Absence of pulse or signs of life.
  - Unresponsiveness, apnea, or gasping.
  - Cyanosis.
- Management:
  - Start CPR immediately.
  - Use age-appropriate defibrillation if indicated.
  - Administer medications per PALS (Pediatric

Advanced Life Support) guidelines.
- ○ Consider underlying causes (e.g., hypovolemia, respiratory failure).

3. Seizures:

- Recognition:
    - ○ Convulsions, loss of consciousness.
    - ○ Abnormal eye movements, staring, or rhythmic movements.
    - ○ Postictal state.
- Management:
    - ○ Ensure a safe environment.
    - ○ Protect the airway.
    - ○ Administer antiepileptic medications as prescribed.
    - ○ Consider emergency medications if seizures persist.

4. Shock:

- Recognition:
    - ○ Tachycardia, weak or absent peripheral pulses.
    - ○ Hypotension, cool extremities.
    - ○ Altered mental status.
- Management:
    - ○ Assess and address the underlying cause (e.g., hypovolemia, sepsis).
    - ○ Provide fluid resuscitation.
    - ○ Consider vasoactive medications.

5. Dehydration:

- Recognition:
    - ○ Decreased urine output, and dry mucous membranes.
    - ○ Sunken fontanelle in infants.

- ○ Irritability, lethargy.
- Management:
  - ○ Rehydration with oral or intravenous fluids.
  - ○ Monitor electrolyte imbalances.
  - ○ Identify and treat the underlying cause (e.g., gastroenteritis).

6. Anaphylaxis:

- Recognition:
  - ○ Rapid onset of hives, itching, swelling.
  - ○ Respiratory distress, wheezing.
  - ○ Hypotension, confusion.
- Management:
  - ○ Administer epinephrine promptly.
  - ○ Secure the airway if necessary.
  - ○ Provide supportive care (e.g., antihistamines, corticosteroids).

7. Sepsis:

- Recognition:
  - ○ Fever or hypothermia.
  - ○ Tachycardia, tachypnea.
  - ○ Altered mental status.
  - ○ Signs of poor perfusion.
- Management:
  - ○ Administer broad-spectrum antibiotics.
  - ○ Provide fluid resuscitation.
  - ○ Monitor for signs of shock.
  - ○ Identify and treat the source of infection.

8. Trauma:

- Recognition:

- Visible injuries, and deformities.
- Altered mental status.
- Signs of internal bleeding (e.g., ecchymosis, abdominal distension).

- Management:
  - Stabilize the cervical spine if trauma is suspected.
  - Control bleeding.
  - Administer pain management.
  - Arrange for appropriate imaging studies.

9. Foreign Body Aspiration:

- Recognition:
  - Sudden onset of coughing, and choking.
  - Stridor, wheezing, or decreased breath sounds.
  - Cyanosis.
- Management:
  - Perform back blows and chest thrusts in infants.
  - Abdominal thrusts in older children.
  - Be prepared for advanced airway intervention if needed.

10. Burns:

- Recognition:
  - Redness, blistering, or charring of the skin.
  - Pain, swelling.
- Management:
  - Cool the burn with running water.
  - Remove clothing around the burn area.
  - Administer pain management.
  - Consider fluid resuscitation for severe burns.

General Principles for Pediatric Emergency Management:

1. **Early Recognition:**
   - Promptly recognize signs of distress or deterioration.
   - Be vigilant for subtle signs in pediatric patients.
2. **Effective Communication:**
   - communicate with parents, guardians, and other healthcare team members.
   - Provide regular updates on the child's condition.
3. **Age-Appropriate Interventions:**
   - Consider age-specific anatomy, physiology, and medication dosages.
   - Use size-appropriate equipment.
4. **Family-Centered Care:**
   - Involve parents in decision-making.
   - Provide emotional support and information to families.
5. **Team Collaboration:**
   - Work collaboratively with the healthcare team.
   - delegate tasks during emergencies.
6. **Continuous Monitoring:**
   - Continuously monitor vital signs and responses to interventions.
   - Be prepared to adjust management based on changes in the patient's condition.
7. **Documentation:**
   - Accurately document assessments, interventions, and responses.
   - Ensure thorough handovers during transitions of care.
8. **Training and Simulation:**
   - Regularly train and simulate pediatric emergency scenarios.
   - Promote ongoing education for healthcare

providers.

Remember that pediatric emergencies can be emotionally challenging for both healthcare providers and families. A compassionate and empathetic approach is essential in providing optimal care during these critical situations.

CPR and Basic Life Support for Children

Cardiopulmonary Resuscitation (CPR) and Basic Life Support (BLS) for children involve a set of life-saving techniques designed to maintain blood circulation and provide oxygen to vital organs in case of cardiac arrest or respiratory failure. Performing CPR and BLS promptly can significantly improve the chances of survival for a child in an emergency. Here are the key steps for CPR and BLS for children:

1. Assess the Situation:

- Ensure the safety of both the child and yourself.
- Check for responsiveness by tapping the child and shouting.
- If unresponsive, shout for help.

2. Activate Emergency Medical Services (EMS):

- Call for emergency help or instruct someone to call.
- Provide specific information about the child's condition and location.

3. Check for Breathing:

- Open the child's airway by tilting the head back and lifting the chin.
- Look, listen, and feel for breathing for no more than 10 seconds.
- If not breathing normally, begin CPR.

4. Chest Compressions:

- Position the child on a firm surface.
- Place the heel of one hand on the center of the chest (just below the nipple line).
- Use both hands for compressions, keeping fingers off the chest.

- Compress the chest at least 2 inches deep at a rate of 100-120 compressions per minute.
- Allow for complete chest recoil between compressions.

5. Rescue Breaths:

- After 30 compressions, provide 2 rescue breaths.
- Ensure a good seal over the child's mouth and nose.
- Deliver each breath over 1 second, with enough volume to make the chest rise visibly.
- Avoid excessive ventilation to prevent gastric inflation.

6. Continue CPR Cycle:

- Perform cycles of 30 compressions and 2 rescue breaths.
- Continue until the child starts breathing on their own, emergency medical help arrives, or you are too exhausted to continue.

7. Automated External Defibrillator (AED):

- If an AED is available, use it as soon as possible.
- Follow the AED prompts for pad placement and operation.
- Resume CPR immediately after AED shock delivery.

8. Child-Specific Considerations:

- **Depth of Compressions:** Compress the chest at least one-third of the depth of the chest, approximately 2 inches for most children.
- **Ventilation:** Ensure effective ventilation without excessive force.
- **Two-Rescuer CPR:** If another trained rescuer is available, consider switching roles every 2 minutes to prevent fatigue.

9. Choking in a Responsive Child:

- Encourage the child to cough if they can.
- If the child is unable to cough, perform back blows and

abdominal thrusts until the object is expelled or emergency help arrives.

10. Choking in an Unresponsive Child:

- Begin CPR immediately, incorporating chest compressions and rescue breaths.
- Check for visible foreign objects during each cycle and remove them if seen.

11. Recovery Position:

- If the child is breathing but unconscious, place them in a recovery position to maintain an open airway.
- Monitor for changes in condition.

12. Continuous Assessment:

- Regularly reassess the child's breathing and responsiveness.
- Adjust interventions based on the child's condition.

Remember:

- Ensure proper hand placement and compression depth during chest compressions.
- Minimize interruptions during CPR to maintain blood flow.

Certification and Training:

- CPR and BLS training is essential for anyone likely to provide care for children.
- Certification courses, such as Pediatric Basic Life Support (PBLS) or Pediatric Advanced Life Support (PALS), are available and provide comprehensive training.

Seek Professional Assistance:

- Always seek professional medical assistance as soon as

possible.

- Continue CPR until professional help arrives or the child starts breathing on their own.

Being prepared to perform CPR and BLS for children is crucial, and regular training ensures that individuals are equipped with the skills needed during emergencies. Certified courses also cover specific pediatric techniques and considerations, helping healthcare providers and caregivers respond effectively to a child in distress.

Chapter 8

Nutritional Needs in Children

Nutrition plays a crucial role in the growth, development, and overall health of children. Meeting the nutritional needs of children is essential for optimal physical and cognitive development. Here are key aspects of nutritional needs in children:

1. Macronutrients:

- Protein:
  - Essential for growth, tissue repair, and immune function.
  - Good sources: lean meats, poultry, fish, dairy products, legumes, nuts, and seeds.
- Carbohydrates:
  - Provide energy for daily activities and brain function.
  - Good sources: whole grains, fruits, vegetables, and legumes.
- Fats:
  - Important for brain development, energy, and absorption of fat-soluble vitamins.
  - Include healthy fats from sources like avocados, nuts, seeds, and olive oil.

2. Micronutrients:

- Vitamins:
  - **Vitamin A:** Essential for vision, immune function, and skin health. Found in sweet potatoes, carrots, spinach, and dairy.
  - **Vitamin C:** Supports immune function and helps the body absorb iron. Found in citrus fruits, strawberries, and bell peppers.
  - **Vitamin D:** Important for bone health and immune function. Sources include fortified dairy, fatty fish, and sunlight.

- ◦ **Vitamin E:** Antioxidant that protects cells. Found in nuts, seeds, and vegetable oils.
- **Minerals:**
  - ◦ **Calcium:** Crucial for bone and teeth development. Found in dairy products, leafy greens, and fortified foods.
  - ◦ **Iron:** Essential for preventing anemia and supporting cognitive development. Found in lean meats, beans, and fortified cereals.
  - ◦ **Zinc:** Important for growth and immune function. Sources include meat, dairy, and whole grains.

3. Proper Hydration:

- Water is essential for various bodily functions, including digestion, nutrient transport, and temperature regulation.
- Encourage children to drink water regularly, especially during physical activity.

4. Balanced Diet:

- Encourage a variety of foods to ensure a balance of nutrients.
- Include fruits, vegetables, whole grains, lean proteins, and dairy or dairy alternatives in meals.

5. Energy Requirements:

- Children have varying energy needs based on factors like age, gender, growth rate, and physical activity level.
- Ensure an appropriate balance between energy intake and expenditure to support growth.

6. Breastfeeding and Infant Nutrition:

- Breastfeeding is recommended for the first six months of life, followed by the introduction of complementary foods.
- Infant formulas provide necessary nutrients for formula-fed infants.
- Introduce solid foods around 6 months, starting with iron-

rich foods.

7. Adolescent Nutrition:

- Adolescents experience rapid growth and have increased nutritional needs.
- Emphasize the importance of a balanced diet, including calcium for bone health and iron for growth.

8. Special Considerations:

- **Food Allergies:** Be aware of and manage food allergies by avoiding trigger foods.
- **Vegetarian or Vegan Diets:** Ensure adequate intake of essential nutrients such as protein, iron, calcium, vitamin B12, and omega-3 fatty acids.
- **Picky Eaters:** Encourage a variety of foods and involve children in meal preparation to make the experience enjoyable.

9. Limiting Sugars and Processed Foods:

- Limit the intake of sugary beverages, snacks, and processed foods.
- Encourage whole, minimally processed foods.

10. Meal Timing and Regular Eating:

- Encourage regular meals and snacks to provide a steady source of energy.
- Promote family meals as an opportunity for socialization and healthy eating habits.

11. Nutritional Education:

- Teach children about the importance of nutrition and making healthy food choices.
- Involve them in grocery shopping and meal preparation.

12. Monitoring Growth and Development:

- Regularly monitor a child's growth and development.
- Consult with healthcare professionals for guidance on nutritional needs and any concerns.

13. Hygiene and Food Safety:

- Emphasize the importance of hygiene during food preparation and consumption.
- Teach children about proper handwashing and food safety practices.

14. Encourage Physical Activity:

- Combine a healthy diet with regular physical activity to support overall well-being.

15. Seek Professional Guidance:

- Consult with pediatricians or registered dietitians for personalized advice, especially for children with specific dietary needs or medical conditions.

Meeting the nutritional needs of children is a collaborative effort involving parents, caregivers, educators, and healthcare professionals. By providing a well-balanced diet, fostering healthy eating habits, and promoting a positive food environment, children can develop into healthy individuals with optimal growth and development.

Age-Appropriate Nutrition

Age-appropriate nutrition is crucial for promoting optimal growth, development, and overall health at different stages of life. Nutrient requirements vary across infancy, childhood, adolescence, and adulthood. Here are guidelines for age-appropriate nutrition:

Infancy (0-12 months):

1. **Breastfeeding or Formula Feeding:**
   - Breastfeeding is recommended for the first six months of life.
   - Infant formula is a suitable alternative when breastfeeding is not possible.
   - Introduce iron-fortified infant cereals around 6 months.
2. **Introduction of Solid Foods:**
   - Begin introducing single-ingredient pureed fruits, vegetables, and iron-fortified cereals around 6 months.
   - Gradually introduce a variety of foods while monitoring for potential allergies.
3. **Avoid Added Sugars and Salt:**
   - Limit or avoid added sugars and salt in infant foods.
4. **Encourage Self-Feeding:**
   - Introduce finger foods and encourage self-feeding to develop fine motor skills.
5. **Supplement with Vitamin D:**
   - Consider a vitamin D supplement, as breast milk is low in this vitamin.

Early Childhood (1-5 years):

1. **Balanced Meals:**

- Provide a variety of foods from all food groups, including fruits, vegetables, whole grains, lean proteins, and dairy.

2. **Portion Sizes:**
   - Adjust portion sizes to meet the child's energy needs and promote healthy growth.

3. **Limit Sugary Beverages:**
   - Limit the consumption of sugary drinks and encourage water.
   - Choose whole fruits over fruit juices.

4. **Calcium-Rich Foods:**
   - Ensure an adequate intake of calcium for bone development through dairy or fortified alternatives.

5. **Snack Choices:**
   - Offer healthy snacks, such as fruits, vegetables, yogurt, and whole grain crackers.

6. **Model Healthy Eating:**
   - Be a role model for healthy eating habits.

Middle Childhood (6-12 years):

1. **Varied Diet:**
   - Continue to offer a diverse range of foods to meet nutrient needs.
   - Emphasize whole foods over processed snacks.

2. **Increased Independence:**
   - Encourage children to make healthy food choices and develop independence in meal preparation.

3. **Mindful Eating:**
   - Encourage mindful eating, paying attention to hunger and fullness cues.

4. **Balanced Meals:**
   - Include protein-rich foods, whole grains, fruits,

vegetables, and healthy fats in meals.

5. **Limit Processed Foods:**
   - Reduce the intake of highly processed and sugary foods.

6. **Hydration:**
   - Ensure an adequate intake of water.
   - Limit sugary beverages.

Adolescence (13-18 years):

1. **Nutrient-Dense Diet:**
   - Emphasize nutrient-dense foods to support rapid growth and development.
   - Include lean proteins, whole grains, fruits, vegetables, and dairy or alternatives.

2. **Calcium and Vitamin D:**
   - Ensure sufficient calcium and vitamin D for bone health.
   - Encourage dairy, fortified plant-based alternatives, and exposure to sunlight.

3. **Iron-Rich Foods:**
   - Promote iron-rich foods to support increased blood volume during puberty.
   - Include lean meats, beans, lentils, and fortified cereals.

4. **Healthy Snacking:**
   - Encourage healthy snacks, such as nuts, seeds, fruits, and yogurt.

5. **Limit Added Sugars and Processed Foods:**
   - Be mindful of added sugars in beverages and processed foods.
   - Encourage whole, minimally processed foods.

6. **Hydration:**

- Emphasize the importance of staying hydrated, especially during physical activities.

7. **Address Individual Nutritional Needs:**
   - Consider individual needs and preferences, including dietary restrictions or preferences.

Adulthood (19 years and older):

1. **Balanced Diet:**
   - Maintain a well-balanced diet with a variety of foods.
   - Adjust portion sizes based on activity level and energy needs.

2. **Nutrient-Rich Choices:**
   - Choose nutrient-dense foods to meet nutritional requirements.

3. **Fiber Intake:**
   - Include fiber-rich foods for digestive health, such as whole grains, fruits, vegetables, and legumes.

4. **Limit Saturated and Trans Fats:**
   - Limit intake of saturated and trans fats.
   - Choose healthy fats from sources like avocados, nuts, and olive oil.

5. **Hydration:**
   - Continue to prioritize hydration with water as the main beverage.

6. **Calcium and Vitamin D:**
   - Maintain adequate calcium and vitamin D intake for bone health.

7. **Monitor Sodium Intake:**
   - Be mindful of sodium intake by limiting processed and high-sodium foods.

8. **Regular Physical Activity:**

- Pair a healthy diet with regular physical activity to support overall well-being.

9. **Regular Health Check-ups:**
   - Attend regular health check-ups to monitor nutritional status and address any concerns.

Individual nutritional needs can vary, and it's essential to consider factors such as health conditions, lifestyle, and personal preferences. Consulting with a registered dietitian or healthcare professional can provide personalized guidance based on specific needs and goals at different life stages.

Breastfeeding and Formula Feeding

Breastfeeding and formula feeding are two methods of providing infants with the essential nutrients they need for growth and development. Each method has its advantages and considerations, and the choice between breastfeeding and formula feeding is a personal decision that depends on various factors. Here's an overview of both approaches:

Breastfeeding:

Advantages:

1. **Nutrient Composition:**
   - Breast milk is uniquely tailored to the nutritional needs of the baby and changes in composition as the baby grows.
   - Provides antibodies and immune factors, offering protection against infections.
2. **Digestibility:**
   - Easily digested, reducing the likelihood of constipation and digestive issues.
3. **Bonding and Comfort:**
   - Promotes bonding between the mother and baby.
   - Provides comfort and a sense of security for the baby.
4. **Reduced Risk of Infections:**
   - Reduces the risk of ear infections, respiratory infections, and gastrointestinal infections in infants.
5. **Maternal Health Benefits:**
   - Promotes uterine contractions, aiding in postpartum recovery.
   - May reduce the risk of breast and ovarian cancers in mothers.

6. **Cost:**
   - Breast milk is free, eliminating the cost of formula.

Considerations:

1. **Time and Commitment:**
   - Requires time and commitment from the mother, especially in the early months.
2. **Maternal Health Considerations:**
   - Maternal health, diet, and lifestyle can impact the quality of breast milk.
3. **Logistics:**
   - May require planning and accommodations for breastfeeding in public places or workplaces.
4. **Potential Challenges:**
   - Some mothers may experience challenges such as breastfeeding difficulties, latch issues, or low milk supply.

Formula Feeding:
Advantages:

1. **Flexibility:**
   - Allows for shared feeding responsibilities between parents and caregivers.
   - Provides flexibility in feeding schedules.
2. **Quantifiable Intake:**
   - Allows caregivers to know precisely how much the baby is eating.
3. **Maternal Independence:**
   - Enables the mother to share feeding responsibilities, allowing more independence.
4. **Nutritional Consistency:**
   - Formula provides a consistent nutritional profile,

irrespective of maternal health or diet.

5. **Easier for Some Mothers:**
   - Can be a preferable option for mothers who face challenges with breastfeeding.

Considerations:

1. **Cost:**
   - Formula feeding incurs the cost of purchasing formula and related supplies.
2. **Preparation and Cleaning:**
   - Formula preparation requires time for measuring, mixing, and sterilizing equipment.
3. **Lack of Immune Protection:**
   - Formula-fed infants may miss some of the immune protection provided by breast milk.
4. **Increased Risk of Infections:**
   - Formula-fed infants may have a slightly higher risk of certain infections compared to breastfed infants.
5. **Storage and Handling:**
   - Prepared formula requires proper storage and handling to ensure safety.

Combination Feeding (Mixed Feeding):

Some parents choose to combine breastfeeding and formula feeding, providing both breast milk and formula based on individual circumstances and preferences. This approach can offer a balance between the benefits of breast milk and the flexibility of formula.

Important Considerations:

1. **Feeding on Demand:**
   - Respond to the baby's hunger cues and feed on demand.
2. **Responsive Feeding:**

- Encourage responsive feeding, allowing the baby to eat until satisfied.

3. **Consultation with Healthcare Professionals:**
   - Discuss feeding choices with healthcare providers for personalized guidance.

4. **Maternal Well-being:**
   - Prioritize the mother's well-being and mental health when making feeding decisions.

Ultimately, the decision between breastfeeding and formula feeding depends on individual circumstances, including maternal preferences, health considerations, and the baby's needs. Both methods can contribute to a baby's healthy growth and development when approached with care and attention to the baby's cues and nutritional needs. Consulting with healthcare professionals can provide valuable guidance and support in making informed decisions.

Childhood Obesity Prevention

Preventing childhood obesity is a multifaceted challenge that involves promoting healthy lifestyle habits at home, in schools, and within communities. Here are key strategies for preventing childhood obesity:

1. Promote Healthy Eating Habits:

- **Balanced Diet:** Encourage a balanced diet that includes fruits, vegetables, whole grains, lean proteins, and low-fat dairy.
- **Limit Sugary Beverages:** Reduce the consumption of sugary drinks and encourage water, milk, or other low-calorie options.
- **Family Meals:** Promote regular family meals, providing an opportunity for healthy eating and positive social interactions.

2. Encourage Regular Physical Activity:

- **Daily Exercise:** Aim for at least 60 minutes of moderate to vigorous physical activity per day for children.
- **Limit Screen Time:** Restrict screen time, including television, computer, and video games, to less than two hours per day.
- **Outdoor Play:** Encourage outdoor play and recreational activities to promote physical fitness.

3. Support Breastfeeding:

- Encourage and support breastfeeding, as it has been linked to a lower risk of childhood obesity.
- Promote breastfeeding-friendly environments in communities and workplaces.

4. Create Healthy Environments:

- **Access to Healthy Foods:** Increase access to affordable, nutritious foods in communities, particularly in areas with limited grocery store access (food deserts).
- **Safe Spaces for Play:** Create safe environments that encourage physical activity, such as parks and playgrounds.
- **Walkable Communities:** Design communities that support walking and biking.

5. Promote Nutrition Education:

- **School Programs:** Implement nutrition education programs in schools that teach children about healthy food choices and the importance of physical activity.
- **Parental Involvement:** Involve parents in nutrition education initiatives, providing them with resources and information.

6. Monitor and Limit Advertising of Unhealthy Foods:

- Advocate for policies that limit the advertising of unhealthy foods and beverages to children.
- Promote positive messages about healthy eating in media campaigns.

7. Early Intervention:

- Monitor children's growth and intervene early if there are signs of excessive weight gain.
- Provide support and resources for families to address obesity risk factors.

8. School Wellness Policies:

- Encourage the development and implementation of comprehensive school wellness policies that address nutrition, physical activity, and overall health.
- Ensure access to healthy food options in school cafeterias.

9. Involve Healthcare Professionals:

- Healthcare providers should routinely monitor children's growth and guide healthy lifestyle habits during well-child visits.
- Address obesity-related concerns with a holistic approach, involving nutritionists, psychologists, and other professionals as needed.

10. Family Engagement:

- Involve families in obesity prevention efforts, providing resources and information on healthy living.
- Encourage positive role modeling by parents and caregivers.

11. Policy Advocacy:

- Advocate for policies at the local, state, and national levels that support healthy eating and physical activity in schools and communities.
- Support policies that improve food labeling and promote transparency.

12. Culturally Tailored Approaches:

- Consider cultural factors when developing obesity prevention strategies, ensuring that interventions are culturally sensitive and relevant.

13. Community Partnerships:

- Build partnerships between schools, healthcare providers, local governments, and community organizations to create a comprehensive approach to childhood obesity prevention.

14. Regular Health Check-ups:

- Ensure regular health check-ups for children, allowing for early identification of potential health issues, including obesity.

15. Empower Children:

- Teach children about the benefits of healthy living and

involve them in decision-making regarding food choices and physical activities.

Preventing childhood obesity requires a collaborative effort involving families, schools, healthcare professionals, policymakers, and communities. By implementing comprehensive strategies that address multiple factors influencing children's health, it is possible to create environments that support healthy lifestyles and reduce the risk of childhood obesity.

Chapter 9

Child Abuse and Neglect

Child abuse and neglect are serious issues that can have profound and long-lasting effects on a child's physical, emotional, and psychological well-being. It's important to understand the different forms of child maltreatment, recognize signs of abuse and neglect, and take steps to prevent and address these situations.

Types of Child Maltreatment:

1. **Physical Abuse:**
   - Involves causing harm or injury to a child through actions such as hitting, shaking, burning, or other forms of physical harm.
   - Signs may include unexplained bruises, fractures, or injuries inconsistent with the given explanation.

2. **Emotional Abuse:**
   - Involves the chronic emotional maltreatment of a child, including humiliation, rejection, or verbal abuse.
   - Signs may include extreme behavior, withdrawal, or development of emotional disorders.

3. **Sexual Abuse:**
   - Involves any sexual activity with a child, including molestation, rape, or exposure to sexual content.
   - Signs may include changes in behavior, inappropriate sexual knowledge, or physical symptoms.

4. **Neglect:**
   - Involves the failure to provide for a child's basic needs, such as food, shelter, medical care, supervision, and emotional support.
   - Signs may include poor hygiene, malnutrition,

untreated medical issues, or lack of appropriate supervision.

5. **Child Exploitation:**
    ◦ Involves using a child for personal or financial gain, including child labor, trafficking, or involvement in criminal activities.
    ◦ Signs may include a child's sudden involvement in inappropriate or dangerous activities.

Signs of Child Abuse and Neglect:

1. **Physical Signs:**
    ◦ Unexplained injuries, bruises, burns, or fractures.
    ◦ Delayed physical development or failure to thrive.
    ◦ Consistent hunger or inappropriate dress for the weather.

2. **Behavioral Signs:**
    ◦ Sudden changes in behavior, mood swings, or extreme aggression.
    ◦ Withdrawal from normal activities, fear of certain individuals, or reluctance to go home.
    ◦ Regressive behaviors, such as bedwetting or thumb-sucking.

3. **Emotional Signs:**
    ◦ Low self-esteem, depression, anxiety, or suicidal thoughts.
    ◦ Inappropriate emotional responses to situations.

4. **Cognitive Signs:**
    ◦ Delayed development, learning difficulties, or poor academic performance.
    ◦ Difficulty forming healthy relationships or trust issues.

5. **Social Signs:**

- ○ Isolation from peers, inability to make friends, or difficulty interacting socially.
- ○ Engaging in high-risk behaviors or substance abuse.

Prevention and Intervention:

1. **Education and Awareness:**
   - ○ Raise awareness about the signs of child abuse and neglect within communities, schools, and healthcare settings.
   - ○ Provide education on positive parenting techniques and stress management.

2. **Parental Support Programs:**
   - ○ Implement programs that provide support and resources to parents, addressing stressors that may contribute to abuse or neglect.

3. **Community Resources:**
   - ○ Ensure access to community resources such as mental health services, counseling, and parenting classes.
   - ○ Establish helplines and hotlines for reporting suspected abuse.

4. **Child Advocacy Centers:**
   - ○ Establish child advocacy centers that coordinate services for abused children, including medical care, counseling, and legal support.

5. **Professional Training:**
   - ○ Provide training for professionals in education, healthcare, and social services to recognize and report signs of abuse.
   - ○ Encourage open communication and collaboration among professionals involved in child welfare.

6. **Legislation and Policies:**

- Advocate for and enforce legislation and policies that protect children from abuse and neglect.
- Strengthen child protective services and ensure adequate funding.

7. **Crisis Intervention:**
   - Develop crisis intervention services to provide immediate support to families in crisis.
   - Ensure swift and appropriate legal intervention in severe cases.

8. **Parental and Community Involvement:**
   - Encourage parental involvement in schools and communities to strengthen support networks.
   - Foster a sense of community responsibility for the well-being of all children.

9. **Trauma-Informed Care:**
   - Implement trauma-informed care approaches in various settings to support children who have experienced abuse and neglect.

10. **Counseling and Therapy:**
    - Provide accessible mental health services for both children and parents to address the emotional consequences of abuse.
    - Offer therapeutic interventions to help families heal and develop healthier coping mechanisms.

Reporting:

If you suspect child abuse or neglect, it is crucial to report your concerns to the appropriate authorities. Reporting procedures vary by location, but generally, you can contact local child protective services, law enforcement, or a child abuse hotline. Remember that reporting is a crucial step in ensuring the safety and well-being of the child.

Child abuse and neglect are serious societal issues that require a comprehensive and collaborative approach. By raising awareness, providing support, and intervening promptly, communities can work toward preventing child maltreatment and creating safer environments for all children.

Identifying Signs of Abuse or Neglect

Identifying signs of abuse or neglect is crucial for the well-being and safety of children. It's essential to be vigilant and aware of potential indicators, as they can vary depending on the type of abuse or neglect. Here are signs associated with different forms of child maltreatment:

Physical Abuse:

1. **Unexplained Injuries:**
   - Frequent bruises, welts, or cuts that are inconsistent with the child's explanation.
   - Injuries in various stages of healing.
2. **Patterned Injuries:**
   - Injuries with distinctive patterns, such as belt marks or handprints.
3. **Unexplained Fractures:**
   - Frequent bone fractures or breaks.
4. **Fear of Physical Contact:**
   - Fear of physical contact or flinching when approached.

Emotional Abuse:

1. **Low Self-Esteem:**
   - Low self-esteem, lack of confidence, or a negative self-image.
2. **Extreme Behavior:**
   - Extreme behavior, such as aggression or withdrawal.
3. **Delayed Development:**
   - Delayed emotional or intellectual development.
4. **Avoidance of Certain People:**
   - Avoidance of a particular person or fear of specific situations.

Sexual Abuse:

1. **Behavioral Changes:**
   - Sudden and unexplained changes in behavior or personality.
2. **Inappropriate Sexual Knowledge:**
   - Possession of knowledge about sexual acts beyond their developmental level.
3. **Sexual Behaviors:**
   - Engaging in explicit sexual behaviors or playing with toys that involve sexual acts.
4. **Genital Pain or Irritation:**
   - Pain, itching, or irritation in the genital area.
5. **Fear of Specific Individuals:**
   - Fear or avoidance of specific individuals.

Neglect:

1. **Malnutrition:**
   - Consistent hunger, poor weight gain, or malnutrition.
2. **Poor Hygiene:**
   - Poor personal hygiene, unwashed clothes, or body odor.
3. **Untreated Medical Issues:**
   - Untreated medical or dental issues.
4. **Inappropriate Dress:**
   - Inadequate or inappropriate clothing for the weather.
5. **Lack of Supervision:**
   - Lack of supervision, especially in dangerous situations.
6. **Failure to Thrive:**
   - Failure to thrive or meet developmental milestones.

Child Exploitation:

1. **Involvement in Illegal Activities:**
   - Involvement in illegal activities, such as drug trafficking or theft.
2. **Unexplained Money or Gifts:**
   - Possession of unexplained money, gifts, or expensive items.
3. **Excessive Absences from School:**
   - Excessive absences from school or decline in academic performance.
4. **Isolation from Peers:**
   - Isolation from peers or sudden changes in social circles.

General Signs:

1. **Fearfulness:**
   - Fearfulness, anxiety, or excessive shyness.
2. **Changes in Sleeping or Eating Patterns:**
   - Disruptions in sleeping or eating patterns.
3. **Regression:**
   - Regression to earlier behaviors, such as bedwetting or thumb-sucking.
4. **Chronic Runaway Attempts:**
   - Chronic runaway attempts or a persistent desire to be away from home.
5. **Poor School Performance:**
   - Decline in school performance, lack of interest in activities, or frequent school absences.

What to Do if You Suspect Abuse or Neglect:

1. **Report to Authorities:**
   - If you suspect abuse or neglect, report your concerns

to the appropriate authorities. Contact local child protective services, law enforcement, or a child abuse hotline.

2. **Document and Report:**
   ◦ Document specific observations and details before reporting.

3. **Seek Professional Guidance:**
   ◦ If you are unsure, seek guidance from professionals such as teachers, counselors, or healthcare providers.

4. **Support the Child:**
   ◦ Offer support and reassurance to the child if they disclose abuse or neglect. Let them know it's not their fault.

5. **Encourage Professional Intervention:**
   ◦ Encourage the involvement of professionals, such as counselors or therapists, for both the child and the family.

6. **Follow Reporting Procedures:**
   ◦ Follow the reporting procedures in your jurisdiction and ensure that the child's safety is the top priority.

Remember that identifying signs of abuse or neglect is a responsibility that should be taken seriously. Reporting suspicions promptly can help protect children and ensure they receive the support and intervention needed for their well-being.

Reporting Procedures and Legal Considerations

Reporting procedures for suspected child abuse or neglect vary by jurisdiction, but there are general guidelines that apply in many regions. It's important to understand the legal and ethical considerations when reporting suspicions of child maltreatment. Below are steps and considerations:

1. Immediate Safety Concerns:

- If a child is in immediate danger, call emergency services (911 or the local emergency number) to ensure swift intervention.

2. Contact Local Child Protective Services:

- In non-emergency situations, contact the local child protective services agency. This agency is often a part of the local or state government's Department of Social Services, Department of Children and Family Services, or a similarly named entity.

3. Follow Reporting Laws:

- Familiarize yourself with the reporting laws and requirements in your jurisdiction. Laws regarding mandatory reporting of child abuse or neglect vary, so it's essential to know the specific regulations that apply in your area.

4. Document Your Observations:

- Document your observations and concerns thoroughly before making a report. Include specific details such as dates, times, locations, and the child's statements (if applicable).

5. Maintain Confidentiality:

- Keep the information confidential to the extent possible while still fulfilling your legal obligation to report. Avoid discussing suspicions with others who do not have a professional need to know.

6. Report Promptly:

- Report suspicions promptly. Delays can hinder the ability to investigate and address potential risks to the child.

7. Report Even if Uncertain:

- If you have reasonable suspicion, it is generally better to report, even if you are not certain. Child protective services professionals will conduct investigations to determine the validity of the concerns.

8. Use Appropriate Channels:

- Follow the designated reporting channels in your jurisdiction. This may involve contacting a child abuse hotline, the local child protective services agency, or both.

9. Provide Necessary Information:

- When making a report, provide the necessary information, including the child's name, age, address, and details about the suspected abuse or neglect. Be prepared to share your observations and any other relevant information.

10. Follow Employer Protocols:

- If you are a mandated reporter due to your profession (e.g., teachers, healthcare professionals), follow your employer's protocols for reporting suspicions of child abuse or neglect.

11. Legal Immunity for Good Faith Reporting:

- In many jurisdictions, individuals who make reports of child abuse or neglect in good faith are protected by legal immunity. This means that as long as the report is made honestly and in the best interest of the child, the reporter is protected from legal repercussions.

12. Cooperate with Authorities:

- If contacted by child protective services or law enforcement during an investigation, cooperate fully. Providing accurate information and participating in the investigative process is crucial for the child's safety.

13. Support for the Reporter:

- Employers of mandated reporters often provide support, training, and resources related to reporting. Seek guidance from your employer or supervisor if needed.

14. Seek Legal Advice if Necessary:

- If you have concerns about potential legal implications, seek advice from legal professionals. Attorneys can provide guidance based on the specific laws in your jurisdiction.

15. Follow Up on the Report:

- If appropriate, follow up on the report to ensure that it was received and that appropriate actions are being taken to address the concerns.

It's essential to prioritize the safety and well-being of the child when reporting suspicions of abuse or neglect. The specific procedures and legal considerations may vary, so individuals should be familiar with the regulations in their local jurisdiction. Additionally, consulting with legal professionals or authorities can provide specific guidance based on the laws applicable to your situation.

Chapter 10

Chronic Pediatric Conditions

Chronic pediatric conditions refer to long-term medical conditions that persist throughout childhood and often require ongoing medical management and care. These conditions can affect various aspects of a child's health, development, and daily life. Healthcare providers, families, and caregivers need to work collaboratively to manage these conditions effectively. Here are some common chronic pediatric conditions:

1. Asthma:

- A chronic respiratory condition characterized by inflammation of the airways, leading to symptoms such as wheezing, coughing, and difficulty breathing.
- Management involves medications (inhaled corticosteroids, bronchodilators), trigger avoidance, and asthma action plans.

2. Diabetes Mellitus:

- A chronic condition where the body's ability to regulate blood glucose (sugar) is impaired.
- Types include Type 1 diabetes (autoimmune) and Type 2 diabetes (often associated with lifestyle factors).
- Management involves insulin therapy, blood glucose monitoring, and dietary management.

3. Cystic Fibrosis:

- A genetic disorder that affects the respiratory, digestive, and reproductive systems, leading to thick, sticky mucus production.
- Treatment includes airway clearance techniques, medications, and nutritional support.

4. Epilepsy:

- A neurological disorder characterized by recurrent seizures, which are disruptions in the normal electrical activity of the brain.
- Management may involve antiepileptic medications and lifestyle modifications.

5. Juvenile Idiopathic Arthritis (JIA):

- An autoimmune disorder causing joint inflammation in children.
- Treatment includes medications to control inflammation, physical therapy, and, in some cases, joint injections.

6. Cerebral Palsy:

- A group of neurological disorders affecting movement and muscle coordination.
- Management involves physical and occupational therapy, assistive devices, and sometimes surgical interventions.

7. Attention-Deficit/Hyperactivity Disorder (ADHD):

- A neurodevelopmental disorder characterized by persistent patterns of inattention, hyperactivity, and impulsivity.
- Treatment may include behavioral therapy, psychoeducation, and, in some cases, medication.

8. Autism Spectrum Disorder (ASD):

- A developmental disorder affecting social communication and behavior.
- Early intervention services, behavioral therapy, and educational support are essential components of management.

9. Congenital Heart Defects:

- Structural abnormalities of the heart present at birth.
- Management varies based on the specific defect and may involve medications, surgeries, or other interventions.

10. Genetic Disorders:

- Conditions caused by abnormalities in a child's DNA.
- Management depends on the specific genetic disorder and may involve supportive care, medications, or specialized therapies.

11. Gastrointestinal Disorders:

- Conditions affecting the digestive system, such as inflammatory bowel disease (Crohn's disease, ulcerative colitis) or celiac disease.
- Management may include medications, dietary modifications, and, in some cases, surgery.

12. Sickle Cell Disease:

- A genetic blood disorder characterized by abnormal hemoglobin, leading to red blood cell deformities and increased risk of complications.
- Treatment includes medications, blood transfusions, and supportive care.

13. Spina Bifida:

- A congenital condition where the spinal cord does not develop properly.
- Treatment involves surgical interventions, physical therapy, and management of associated complications.

14. Muscular Dystrophy:

- A group of genetic disorders leading to progressive muscle weakness and degeneration.

- Management includes supportive care, physical therapy, and, in some cases, medications.

15. Chronic Kidney Disease:

- Long-term impairment of kidney function, which can lead to various complications.
- Treatment may involve medications, dietary restrictions, and, in severe cases, kidney transplantation.

16. Chronic Respiratory Conditions (e.g., Bronchopulmonary Dysplasia):

- Conditions affecting the lungs and respiratory system, often stemming from premature birth or other factors.
- Treatment involves medications, respiratory support, and pulmonary rehabilitation.

17. Childhood Cancer:

- Various types of cancer that can affect children, including leukemia, brain tumors, and lymphomas.
- Treatment involves a combination of surgery, chemotherapy, radiation therapy, and supportive care.

18. HIV/AIDS in Children:

- Chronic viral infections affecting the immune system.
- Management includes antiretroviral therapy (ART) and ongoing medical monitoring.

19. Neuromuscular Disorders:

- Conditions affecting the nerves and muscles, such as muscular dystrophy or spinal muscular atrophy.
- Management may include supportive care, physical therapy,

and assistive devices.

20. Obesity:

- Excess body weight can lead to various health complications.
- Management involves lifestyle modifications, dietary changes, and, in some cases, medical interventions.

Holistic Approach to Management:

The management of chronic pediatric conditions often requires a multidisciplinary and holistic approach, involving healthcare professionals, educators, therapists, and support networks. It's crucial to tailor interventions to the specific needs of the child, considering their medical, psychological, and social well-being. Regular monitoring, timely interventions, and ongoing support contribute to improving the quality of life for children with chronic conditions. Family involvement and education also play key roles in successful management.

Chapter 11

Pediatric Nursing in Specialized Settings

Pediatric nursing in specialized settings involves providing nursing care to children with specific healthcare needs in environments that cater to those needs. Specialized settings can include pediatric hospitals, neonatal intensive care units (NICUs), pediatric intensive care units (PICUs), pediatric oncology units, pediatric rehabilitation centers, and other facilities that focus on specific pediatric populations or medical conditions. Here are some areas of specialized pediatric nursing:

1. Neonatal Intensive Care Unit (NICU):

- **Focus:** Premature infants or newborns with critical medical conditions.
- **Nursing Responsibilities:**
  - Monitoring vital signs and respiratory support.
  - Administering medications and nutrition.
  - Providing developmental care for premature infants.
  - Collaborating with a multidisciplinary team.

2. Pediatric Intensive Care Unit (PICU):

- **Focus:** Critically ill children with various medical and surgical conditions.
- **Nursing Responsibilities:**
  - Continuous monitoring of vital signs.
  - Administering medications and interventions.
  - Collaborating with physicians and specialists.
  - Family support and education.

3. Pediatric Cardiac Intensive Care Unit (CICU):

- **Focus:** Children with congenital or acquired heart conditions.
- **Nursing Responsibilities:**
  - Monitoring cardiac status and interventions.
  - Administering medications.
  - Assisting with post-surgical care.

  ○ Educating families on cardiac care.

4. Pediatric Oncology Nursing:

- **Focus:** Children with cancer or hematologic disorders.
- **Nursing Responsibilities:**
  - ○ Administering chemotherapy and supportive care.
  - ○ Monitoring for complications and side effects.
  - ○ Providing emotional support to the child and family.
  - ○ Collaborating with oncology specialists.

5. Pediatric Hematology Nursing:

- **Focus:** Children with blood disorders, such as sickle cell anemia or hemophilia.
- **Nursing Responsibilities:**
  - ○ Administering blood products.
  - ○ Monitoring for complications and managing symptoms.
  - ○ Collaborating with hematologists.

6. Pediatric Neurology Nursing:

- **Focus:** Children with neurological conditions, such as epilepsy or cerebral palsy.
- **Nursing Responsibilities:**
  - ○ Monitoring neurological status.
  - ○ Administering medications.
  - ○ Providing support for families coping with chronic conditions.

7. Pediatric Respiratory Nursing:

- **Focus:** Children with respiratory conditions, such as asthma or cystic fibrosis.
- **Nursing Responsibilities:**
  - ○ Administering respiratory treatments.
  - ○ Monitoring lung function.
  - ○ Educating families on respiratory care.

8. Pediatric Rehabilitation Nursing:

- **Focus:** Children with physical or developmental disabilities.
- **Nursing Responsibilities:**
  - Collaborating with physical and occupational therapists.
  - Assisting with rehabilitation activities.
  - Providing support for families adapting to new challenges.

9. Pediatric Surgical Nursing:

- **Focus:** Children undergoing surgical procedures.
- **Nursing Responsibilities:**
  - Preoperative and postoperative care.
  - Monitoring for complications.
  - Supporting families through the surgical process.

10. Pediatric Home Healthcare Nursing:

- **Focus:** Children receiving healthcare services at home.
- **Nursing Responsibilities:**
  - Administering medications.
  - Monitoring health status.
  - Providing education and support to families.

11. Pediatric Emergency Nursing:

- **Focus:** Acute care for children in emergencies.
- **Nursing Responsibilities:**
  - Rapid assessment and intervention.
  - Stabilizing critically ill or injured children.
  - Collaborating with emergency medicine teams.

12. Pediatric Infectious Disease Nursing:

- **Focus:** Children with infectious diseases, such as HIV or serious bacterial infections.

- Nursing Responsibilities:
  - Administering antimicrobial medications.
  - Implementing infection control measures.
  - Educating families on prevention and management.

13. Pediatric Psychiatry Nursing:

- **Focus:** Children with mental health conditions.
- Nursing Responsibilities:
  - Administering psychiatric medications.
  - Participating in therapeutic interventions.
  - Collaborating with mental health professionals.

14. Pediatric Endocrinology Nursing:

- **Focus:** Children with endocrine disorders, such as diabetes or growth hormone deficiencies.
- Nursing Responsibilities:
  - Administering hormonal therapies.
  - Educating families on managing chronic conditions.
  - Monitoring growth and development.

15. Pediatric Nephrology Nursing:

- **Focus:** Children with kidney disorders or renal failure.
- Nursing Responsibilities:
  - Administering renal replacement therapies.
  - Monitoring fluid and electrolyte balance.
  - Assisting with transplant care.

Key Skills for Pediatric Nurses in Specialized Settings:

1. **Clinical Expertise:** Specialized knowledge and skills related to the specific pediatric population or medical condition.
2. **Effective Communication:** Collaborating with a multidisciplinary team, communicating with children, and providing education to families.

3. **Compassion and Empathy:** Recognizing the unique needs of children and families in specialized settings.
4. **Adaptability:** Managing complex and dynamic healthcare situations that may arise in specialized pediatric care.
5. **Patient and Family Advocacy:** Advocating for the best interests of the child and ensuring that families are informed and supported.
6. **Critical Thinking:** Assessing and managing complex healthcare situations, making sound clinical judgments.
7. **Crisis Management:** Responding effectively to emergencies and rapidly changing situations.
8. **Cultural Competence:** Recognizing and respecting diverse cultural backgrounds and beliefs when providing care.

Pediatric nursing in specialized settings requires a high level of expertise, dedication, and a commitment to providing family-centered care. Nurses in these settings play a vital role in supporting the health and well-being of children facing various medical challenges.

Chapter 12

Psychosocial Issues in Pediatric Care

Pediatric care involves addressing not only the physical health of children but also their psychosocial well-being. Psychosocial issues encompass a wide range of factors that influence a child's mental, emotional, and social development. Healthcare professionals, including pediatric nurses, play a crucial role in identifying and addressing these issues to support the overall health and resilience of children. Here are some key psychosocial issues in pediatric care:

1. Child and Family Adjustment:

- **Issue:** Adapting to a new diagnosis, chronic illness, or treatment plan.
- **Nursing Role:**
    - Provide emotional support to both the child and family.
    - Facilitate open communication about fears and concerns.
    - Offer resources for coping and adjustment.

2. Anxiety and Fear:

- **Issue:** Anxiety related to medical procedures, hospitalization, or unfamiliar healthcare environments.
- **Nursing Role:**
    - Use age-appropriate explanations and preparation.
    - Employ distraction techniques and play therapy.
    - Collaborate with child life specialists for support.

3. Grief and Loss:

- **Issue:** Coping with the loss of normalcy, physical abilities, or the death of a loved one.
- **Nursing Role:**
    - Provide grief support and counseling.
    - Encourage open discussions about loss.
    - Connect families with bereavement resources.

4. School and Developmental Challenges:

- **Issue:** Balancing healthcare needs with academic and developmental milestones.
- **Nursing Role:**
  - Collaborate with educators to support academic accommodations.
  - Advocate for developmental assessments and interventions.
  - Facilitate communication between healthcare and educational teams.

5. Peer Relationships:

- **Issue:** Navigating social interactions and relationships with peers.
- **Nursing Role:**
  - Encourage socialization and inclusion.
  - Address concerns related to self-esteem.
  - Provide strategies for peer education about the child's condition.

6. Parental Stress and Coping:

- **Issue:** Managing stress and coping with the demands of caregiving.
- **Nursing Role:**
  - Assess parental stress levels.
  - Offer support and coping strategies.
  - Connect parents with support groups and counseling services.

7. Cultural and Diversity Considerations:

- **Issue:** Navigating healthcare practices and beliefs that vary across cultures.
- **Nursing Role:**
  - Be culturally competent and sensitive.
  - Incorporate cultural practices into care plans.
  - Seek input from families regarding cultural

preferences.

8. Behavioral and Emotional Disorders:

- **Issue:** Managing behavioral challenges and emotional disorders.

- **Nursing Role:**
  - Collaborate with mental health professionals.
  - Provide behavioral interventions and support.
  - Educate families on available mental health resources.

9. Transition to Adulthood:

- **Issue:** Preparing adolescents for the transition from pediatric to adult healthcare.

- **Nursing Role:**
  - Facilitate discussions about transition planning.
  - Promote self-advocacy and independence.
  - Collaborate with adult healthcare providers.

10. Financial Strain:

- **Issue:** Coping with the financial burden of medical expenses and care.

- **Nursing Role:**
  - Connect families with financial assistance programs.
  - Advocate for resources and support.
  - Provide information on available community resources.

11. Siblings' Needs:

- **Issue:** Addressing the needs and concerns of siblings of children with health challenges.

- **Nursing Role:**
  - Include siblings in discussions and activities when appropriate.
  - Offer sibling support services.
  - Educate families on fostering positive sibling

relationships.

12. Health Literacy:

- **Issue:** Ensuring that families understand medical information and treatment plans.

- **Nursing Role:**
  - Use plain language and visual aids in education.
  - Assess health literacy levels and provide tailored information.
  - Encourage questions and open communication.

13. Trauma and PTSD:

- **Issue:** Coping with the psychological impact of traumatic experiences.

- **Nursing Role:**
  - Identify signs of trauma and PTSD.
  - Collaborate with mental health professionals for support.
  - Implement trauma-informed care approaches.

14. Ethical Dilemmas:

- **Issue:** Navigating complex ethical decisions related to the child's care.

- **Nursing Role:**
  - Engage in ethical discussions with the healthcare team.
  - Advocate for the child's best interests.
  - Provide support to families facing difficult decisions.

15. Technology and Screen Time:

- **Issue:** Balancing the use of technology for medical care with healthy screen time practices.

- **Nursing Role:**
  - Educate families on age-appropriate screen time guidelines.
  - Provide resources for positive screen time habits.

- ○ Monitor and address potential negative impacts.

Strategies for Pediatric Nurses:

1. **Build Trusting Relationships:**
   - ○ Establish trusting relationships with children and families to facilitate open communication.
2. **Provide Family-Centered Care:**
   - ○ Involve families in care planning and decision-making, recognizing their expertise in their child's needs.
3. **Educate and Empower:**
   - ○ Provide clear and understandable information to families, empowering them to actively participate in their child's care.
4. **Collaborate with Multidisciplinary Teams:**
   - ○ Work collaboratively with healthcare professionals from various disciplines to address the diverse needs of the child.
5. **Advocate for Psychosocial Support Services:**
   - ○ Advocate for and facilitate access to psychosocial support services, including counseling, social work, and child life services.
6. **Utilize Developmentally Appropriate Interventions:**
   - ○ Tailor interventions to the developmental stage of the child, considering age-specific needs and preferences.
7. **Promote Resilience:**
   - ○ Support the development of resilience in children and families, emphasizing strengths and coping strategies.
8. **Cultural Competence:**
   - ○ Be culturally competent and sensitive, recognizing

and respecting diverse backgrounds and beliefs.

9. **Trauma-Informed Care:**
    ◦ Implement trauma-informed care approaches to address the impact of past traumatic experiences.

10. **Encourage Peer Support:**
    ◦ Facilitate opportunities for children and families to connect with peer support networks, fostering a sense of community.

11. **Provide Continuity of Care:**
    ◦ Support continuity of care, ensuring that there is consistency in healthcare providers and a seamless transition between healthcare settings.

12. **Offer Follow-Up and Support:**
    ◦ Provide ongoing follow-up and support, recognizing that psychosocial issues may evolve.

Pediatric nurses play a vital role in addressing psychosocial issues to promote the holistic well-being of children and their families. By incorporating these strategies, healthcare professionals can contribute to a supportive and nurturing healthcare environment for pediatric patients

Coping Mechanisms for Children and Families

Coping mechanisms are strategies that individuals use to manage stress, navigate challenges, and adapt to difficult situations. For children and families facing health-related issues, coping mechanisms play a crucial role in promoting resilience and well-being. Pediatric nurses and healthcare professionals can support the development and utilization of effective coping strategies. Here are various coping mechanisms for children and families:

Coping Mechanisms for Children:

1. **Play Therapy:**
   - Utilizing play to help children express emotions, process experiences, and gain a sense of control.
2. **Art and Creative Expression:**
   - Engaging in drawing, painting, or other creative activities as a way to communicate feelings and experiences.
3. **Distraction Techniques:**
   - Using age-appropriate distractions, such as games, toys, or music, to redirect attention during medical procedures or challenging situations.
4. **Storytelling and Narrative:**
   - Encouraging children to share their stories through words, drawings, or role-playing, fostering a sense of self-expression.
5. **Comfort Objects:**
   - Allowing children to have a comfort item, such as a stuffed animal or blanket, for emotional support during medical procedures or hospitalization.
6. **Breathing Exercises:**

- Teaching simple breathing exercises to help children manage anxiety and promote relaxation.

7. **Social Support:**
   - Facilitating connections with friends, family, or support groups to provide a sense of belonging and understanding.

8. **Educational Support:**
   - Involve children in understanding their health conditions through age-appropriate education and information.

9. **Routine and Predictability:**
   - Establishing and maintaining routines to create a sense of stability and predictability.

10. **Positive Imagery:**
    - Guiding children to use their imagination to create positive mental images to counteract negative thoughts.

11. **Therapeutic Play:**
    - Engaging in activities that are both enjoyable and therapeutic, fostering emotional expression and processing.

12. **Music Therapy:**
    - Using music as a tool for relaxation, expression, and emotional release.

Coping Mechanisms for Families:

1. **Open Communication:**
   - Encouraging open and honest communication within the family to share thoughts, concerns, and feelings.

2. **Family Meetings:**
   - Holding regular family meetings to discuss

challenges, plans, and strategies for support.

3. **Collaborative Decision-Making:**
   - Involving family members in decision-making processes related to the child's care and treatment.

4. **Education and Information:**
   - Providing families with accurate and understandable information about the child's condition and treatment.

5. **Parental Support Groups:**
   - Connecting parents with support groups to share experiences, advice, and emotional support.

6. **Respite Care:**
   - Arranging for respite care to give parents a break and time for self-care.

7. **Financial Planning:**
   - Assisting families with financial planning and resources to manage the costs associated with healthcare.

8. **Self-Care for Parents:**
   - Encouraging parents to engage in self-care activities to maintain their own physical and emotional well-being.

9. **Problem-Solving Skills:**
   - Developing problem-solving skills within the family to address challenges collaboratively.

10. **Flexibility and Adaptability:**
    - Encouraging flexibility and adaptability in response to changing circumstances.

11. **Utilizing Extended Support Networks:**
    - Tapping into extended family, friends, and community resources for additional support.

12. **Mindfulness and Relaxation Techniques:**

- Introducing mindfulness and relaxation practices to help manage stress and promote emotional well-being.

13. **Counseling Services:**
    - Offering access to counseling services for individual or family therapy to address emotional and relational challenges.

14. **Celebrating Achievements:**
    - Acknowledging and celebrating milestones and achievements, no matter how small.

15. **Advocacy Skills:**
    - Empowering families to advocate for their child's needs within the healthcare system and community.

Collaborative Approaches:

1. **Team-Based Support:**
    - Involving a multidisciplinary team, including nurses, social workers, child life specialists, and therapists, to provide comprehensive support.

2. **Family-Centered Care:**
    - Embracing a family-centered care approach that involves families as partners in the child's care.

3. **Crisis Intervention:**
    - Implementing crisis intervention strategies during challenging times to provide immediate support.

4. **Long-Term Planning:**
    - Collaborating with families on long-term care plans and goals for the child's health and development.

5. **Advocating for Resources:**
    - Assisting families in accessing community resources, financial assistance, and educational support.

6. **Creating Safe Spaces:**

- Designing environments, both at home and in healthcare settings, that foster a sense of safety and comfort.

7. **Regular Assessments:**
   - Conducting regular assessments of coping mechanisms to identify evolving needs and provide tailored support.

8. **Promoting Empowerment:**
   - Empowering both children and families to actively participate in their healthcare decisions and navigate challenges.

It's important to recognize that coping mechanisms may vary based on the child's age, developmental stage, and individual preferences. Additionally, cultural considerations play a significant role in determining effective coping strategies. Tailoring support to the unique needs of each child and family is essential for promoting resilience and well-being in the face of health-related challenges. Pediatric nurses and healthcare professionals play a vital role in guiding and facilitating the development of these coping mechanisms.

Supporting Children with Chronic Illnesses

Supporting children with chronic illnesses requires a comprehensive and compassionate approach that addresses their physical, emotional, and psychosocial needs. Pediatric nurses, along with a multidisciplinary healthcare team, play a crucial role in providing this support. Here are key strategies for supporting children with chronic illnesses:

1. Education and Information:

- For Families:
  - Provide families with accurate and understandable information about the child's diagnosis, treatment plan, and prognosis.
  - Offer educational materials and resources to enhance their understanding of the chronic illness.
- For Children:
  - Use age-appropriate language to explain the condition and treatment.
  - Involve children in discussions about their health in a developmentally appropriate manner.

2. Emotional Support:

- For Children:
  - Create a supportive and empathetic environment, addressing the child's emotional needs.
  - Encourage age-appropriate expression of feelings and concerns.
  - Facilitate connections with child life specialists or therapists for emotional support.
- For Families:

- ○ Offer counseling services for parents and siblings to cope with the emotional impact of the chronic illness.
- ○ Establish support groups for families to share experiences and provide mutual support.

3. Empowerment and Involvement:

- For Children:
  - ○ Encourage children to actively participate in their care to foster a sense of control.
  - ○ Support the development of self-advocacy skills as age-appropriate.
- For Families:
  - ○ Involve parents in decision-making processes related to the child's care.
  - ○ Provide opportunities for families to collaborate with the healthcare team on care plans.

4. Psychosocial Support Services:

- For Children:
  - ○ Connect children with psychosocial support services, such as play therapy, art therapy, or music therapy.
- For Families:
  - ○ Offer access to counseling services for the family to address the psychosocial impact of the chronic illness.

5. Pain Management:

- Implement effective pain management strategies, including medications, non-pharmacological interventions, and collaboration with pain specialists.

- Monitor and assess pain levels regularly to adjust the management plan as needed.

6. Holistic Care Planning:

- Develop individualized care plans that address the physical, emotional, and social aspects of the child's well-being.
- Collaborate with specialists, therapists, and educators to create a comprehensive care approach.

7. Transition Planning:

- Start planning for the transition from pediatric to adult healthcare well in advance, considering the unique needs of adolescents with chronic illnesses.
- Involve the child and family in discussions about future healthcare management.

8. School Collaboration:

- Work with educators to create a supportive environment for children with chronic illnesses.
- Develop individualized education plans (IEPs) or 504 plans to address academic and health-related needs.

9. Social Integration:

- Facilitate social interactions and integration for children with chronic illnesses.
- Work with schools and communities to promote inclusion and reduce stigma.

10. Nutritional Support:

- Collaborate with dietitians to ensure that children with chronic illnesses receive appropriate and customized nutritional support.

- Monitor and address nutritional challenges associated with the chronic condition.

11. Family-Centered Care:

- Embrace a family-centered care approach that recognizes the family as an essential part of the healthcare team.
- Involve families in care planning, decision-making, and goal-setting.

12. Advocacy:

- Advocate for the needs of children with chronic illnesses within the healthcare system, educational institutions, and the community.
- Support families in advocating for resources, accommodations, and understanding.

13. Regular Follow-Up and Monitoring:

- Schedule regular follow-up appointments to monitor the child's health status and adjust the care plan as needed.
- Conduct assessments of the child's development, mental health, and overall well-being.

14. Financial Support:

- Provide information about financial assistance programs and resources available to families with children with chronic illnesses.
- Advocate for financial support services within the healthcare system.

15. End-of-Life Care and Bereavement Support:

- If applicable, provide compassionate end-of-life care and support for families facing the loss of a child.

- Offer bereavement services and resources to help families cope with grief.

16. Technology and Telehealth:

- Explore the use of technology and telehealth to enhance communication, monitor health remotely, and provide support to families, especially in situations where regular clinic visits may be challenging.

17. Collaboration with Community Resources:

- Connect families with community resources, support organizations, and advocacy groups related to the specific chronic illness.

18. Cultural Competence:

- Be culturally competent and sensitive to the diverse backgrounds and beliefs of children and families.
- Consider cultural preferences and practices in the care plan.

19. Sibling Support:

- Address the needs of siblings by providing information, and emotional support, and involving them in age-appropriate discussions about chronic illness.

20. Celebrate Achievements:

- Acknowledge and celebrate milestones and achievements, no matter how small, to boost the child's and family's morale.

Key Nursing Skills for Supporting Children with Chronic Illnesses:

1. **Effective Communication:**
   - Build strong communication channels with children and families, ensuring clarity and understanding.
2. **Empathy and Compassion:**
   - Demonstrate empathy and compassion to create a supportive and caring environment.
3. **Pediatric Clinical Expertise:**
   - Possess expertise in pediatric nursing, understanding the unique needs and challenges of children with chronic illnesses.
4. **Advocacy Skills:**
   - Advocate for the needs of children and families within the healthcare system and community.
5. **Collaboration:**
   - Collaborate with a multidisciplinary healthcare team, educators, and community resources to provide holistic care.
6. **Crisis Management:**
   - Be prepared to manage crises and provide immediate support when needed.
7. **Family-Centered Care:**
   - Embrace a family-centered care approach that involves families as active participants in the child's care.
8. **Cultural Competence:**
   - Be culturally competent, respecting and integrating cultural considerations into the care plan.
9. **Trauma-Informed Care:**
   - Implement trauma-informed care approaches to address any potential trauma associated with the chronic illness.
10. **Patient and Family Education:**

○ Provide clear and accessible education to children and families, empowering them to actively participate in care.

Supporting children with chronic illnesses requires ongoing collaboration, flexibility, and a commitment to addressing the unique needs of each child and family. By employing these strategies, pediatric nurses contribute significantly to enhancing the quality of life and well-being of children facing chronic health challenges.

Chapter 13

Community and Public Health Nursing

Community and public health nursing involve providing healthcare services and promoting health within communities rather than in individual healthcare settings. These nursing specialties focus on preventing diseases, promoting health and wellness, and addressing the unique healthcare needs of populations. Here are key aspects of community and public health nursing:

Roles and Responsibilities:

1. **Health Promotion and Education:**
    - Develop and implement health education programs to raise awareness about preventive measures, healthy lifestyles, and disease management within the community.

2. **Disease Prevention:**
    - Conduct screenings, immunizations, and other preventive interventions to reduce the incidence of diseases.

3. **Community Assessment:**
    - Assess the health needs and resources of a community through surveys, interviews, and data analysis to identify priority health issues.

4. **Community Planning:**
    - Collaborate with community members, healthcare professionals, and organizations to develop health plans and interventions tailored to the community's specific needs.

5. **Policy Advocacy:**
    - Advocate for policies that promote health and address social determinants of health at local, regional, and national levels.

6. **Emergency Preparedness:**
   - Develop and implement plans to respond to public health emergencies and disasters, ensuring the safety and well-being of the community.
7. **Home Visits:**
   - Conduct home visits to assess individual and family health needs, provide education, and offer support.
8. **Community Partnerships:**
   - Establish and maintain partnerships with local organizations, schools, government agencies, and community leaders to enhance the overall health of the population.
9. **Population Health Management:**
   - Manage the health of specific populations within the community, addressing common health concerns and implementing targeted interventions.
10. **Environmental Health:**
    - Address environmental factors that impact health, such as air and water quality, housing conditions, and workplace safety.
11. **Maternal and Child Health:**
    - Provide prenatal and postnatal care, child health services, and support to families to ensure the well-being of mothers and children.
12. **Chronic Disease Management:**
    - Develop and implement programs for managing chronic conditions, including diabetes, hypertension, and cardiovascular diseases, within the community.
13. **School Health:**
    - Collaborate with schools to promote health and wellness among students, addressing issues such as

nutrition, physical activity, and mental health.

Key Principles:

1. **Preventive Focus:**
   - Emphasize preventive measures and interventions to reduce the occurrence of diseases and improve overall health.
2. **Community Empowerment:**
   - Engage communities in the decision-making process, empowering them to actively participate in their health promotion and disease prevention.
3. **Cultural Competence:**
   - Understand and respect the cultural diversity within the community to provide culturally competent and sensitive care.
4. **Holistic Approach:**
   - Take a holistic approach to health, considering social, economic, environmental, and cultural factors that influence well-being.
5. **Evidence-Based Practice:**
   - Base nursing interventions on evidence-based practices and research to ensure effective and efficient healthcare delivery.
6. **Advocacy:**
   - Advocate for policies, resources, and initiatives that address the social determinants of health and promote equitable healthcare access.
7. **Collaboration:**
   - Collaborate with various stakeholders, including healthcare professionals, community organizations, policymakers, and residents, to achieve common health goals.

8. **Health Equity:**
    - Work towards reducing health disparities and promoting health equity within the community.

Community Health Nursing Process:

1. **Assessment:**
    - Conduct a thorough assessment of the community's health needs, assets, and challenges.
2. **Diagnosis:**
    - Identify priority health issues and determine the underlying causes and risk factors.
3. **Planning:**
    - Develop a comprehensive plan that includes goals, objectives, and interventions to address the identified health issues.
4. **Implementation:**
    - Implement the planned interventions, collaborating with community members and other stakeholders.
5. **Evaluation:**
    - Evaluate the effectiveness of the interventions and make adjustments as needed to achieve desired health outcomes.

Challenges and Considerations:

1. **Limited Resources:**
    - Work with limited resources and funding to implement effective health programs.
2. **Community Resistance:**
    - Address potential resistance or skepticism from the community by building trust through open communication and collaboration.
3. **Cultural Sensitivity:**

- Be sensitive to cultural differences and norms when developing and implementing health interventions.

4. **Addressing Social Determinants:**
   - Tackle social determinants of health, such as poverty, education, and housing, to create lasting improvements in community health.

5. **Data Collection and Analysis:**
   - Ensure accurate and comprehensive data collection and analysis to inform evidence-based practice.

6. **Interprofessional Collaboration:**
   - Collaborate with professionals from various disciplines, including social work, public health, and education, to address multifaceted health issues.

Community and public health nursing play a vital role in improving the health and well-being of populations. Nurses in these roles contribute to preventing diseases, promoting health equity, and addressing the social determinants of health within communities.

Chapter 14

Cultural Competence in Pediatric Nursing

Cultural competence in pediatric nursing involves the ability to understand, respect, and effectively respond to the diverse cultural backgrounds and beliefs of pediatric patients and their families. It is a crucial aspect of providing high-quality, patient-centered care. Culturally competent pediatric nursing involves recognizing and addressing the impact of cultural factors on health and healthcare, promoting inclusivity, and tailoring care to meet the unique needs of each child and family. Here are key principles and strategies for cultural competence in pediatric nursing:

Principles of Cultural Competence:

1. **Respect for Diversity:**
   - Value and respect the diversity of cultural backgrounds, beliefs, and practices within the pediatric population.
2. **Cultural Awareness:**
   - Develop an awareness of one's own cultural biases and assumptions to avoid stereotyping and promote unbiased care.
3. **Cultural Knowledge:**
   - Acquire knowledge about the cultural backgrounds, customs, traditions, and health beliefs of the diverse populations served.
4. **Patient and Family-Centered Care:**
   - Engage patients and their families as active participants in their care, considering their cultural preferences and perspectives.
5. **Effective Communication:**
   - Use clear and culturally sensitive communication,

considering language preferences, non-verbal cues, and the importance of family involvement.

6. **Individualized Care Plans:**
   - Tailor care plans to the unique cultural, social, and spiritual needs of each child and family.

7. **Inclusivity:**
   - Create an inclusive and welcoming healthcare environment that respects and accommodates diverse cultural practices.

8. **Collaboration and Partnership:**
   - Collaborate with interpreters, cultural liaisons, and community resources to bridge language and cultural gaps.

9. **Cultural Competence Training:**
   - Seek ongoing training and education to enhance cultural competence and stay informed about cultural considerations in healthcare.

Strategies for Cultural Competence in Pediatric Nursing:

1. **Cultural Assessment:**
   - Conduct culturally sensitive assessments to understand the beliefs, values, and practices that may influence the child's health and healthcare decisions.

2. **Language Access:**
   - Ensure access to language interpretation services to facilitate effective communication with non-English-speaking families.

3. **Family-Centered Rounds:**
   - Involve families in patient rounds and decision-making processes, considering their cultural perspectives and preferences.

4. **Culturally Competent Education:**
   - Provide educational materials and information that are culturally relevant and accessible to diverse populations.
5. **Understanding Cultural Taboos:**
   - Be aware of and respect cultural taboos and sensitivities that may affect healthcare decisions and practices.
6. **Flexible Visitation Policies:**
   - Consider flexible visitation policies that accommodate cultural practices and family support systems.
7. **Religious and Spiritual Considerations:**
   - Respect and incorporate religious and spiritual considerations into care plans, including dietary restrictions and rituals.
8. **Cultural Rituals during Care:**
   - Incorporate cultural rituals and practices into care, when possible, to provide comfort and maintain cultural identity.
9. **Awareness of Traditional Healing Practices:**
   - Be aware of traditional healing practices that families may use alongside Western medicine, and collaborate with families to integrate these practices safely.
10. **Cultural Competence in End-of-Life Care:**
    - Recognize and respect diverse cultural beliefs and practices related to end-of-life care, grief, and mourning.
11. **Advocacy for Cultural Needs:**
    - Advocate for the cultural needs of pediatric patients and families within the healthcare system, ensuring

that policies and practices are culturally sensitive.

12. **Cultural Competence in Health Promotion:**
    - Design and implement health promotion initiatives that consider cultural perspectives on wellness and preventive care.

13. **Regular Cultural Competence Training:**
    - Engage in regular training sessions on cultural competence to stay informed about evolving cultural considerations in healthcare.

14. **Feedback and Continuous Improvement:**
    - Seek feedback from patients and families about their cultural experiences and use this information for continuous improvement in cultural competence.

15. **Cultural Competence in Pediatric Emergency Care:**
    - Consider cultural factors in emergency care situations, understanding that cultural beliefs may influence decision-making and responses to emergencies.

Challenges and Considerations:

1. **Language Barriers:**
    - Overcoming language barriers to ensure effective communication and understanding.

2. **Cultural Stereotypes:**
    - Avoiding cultural stereotypes and assumptions that may impact the quality of care.

3. **Limited Cultural Competence Resources:**
    - Addressing challenges related to limited resources and training in cultural competence within healthcare settings.

4. **Family Dynamics:**
    - Understanding and respecting diverse family

structures and dynamics.

5. **Cultural Awareness of Pediatric Staff:**
   - Ensuring that pediatric healthcare staff are culturally aware and competent in their interactions.

6. **Cultural Variability:**
   - Recognizing the variability within cultural groups and avoiding generalizations.

7. **Integration of Traditional and Western Medicine:**
   - Navigating the integration of traditional healing practices with Western medicine in a way that respects both approaches.

Cultural competence is an ongoing process that involves self-reflection, continuous learning, and adaptation to the evolving needs of diverse populations. Pediatric nurses play a vital role in fostering cultural competence within healthcare settings, ultimately contributing to improved patient outcomes and satisfaction.

Chapter 15

Ethical and Legal Issues in Pediatric Nursing

Pediatric nursing, like any other area of healthcare, involves complex ethical and legal considerations. Pediatric nurses must navigate these issues to ensure the well-being of their young patients while upholding ethical principles and adhering to legal standards. Here are some key ethical and legal issues in pediatric nursing:

Ethical Issues:

1. **Autonomy of the Child:**
   - Balancing the autonomy of the child with the parental authority, especially in situations where the child may have differing views on treatment options.
2. **Informed Consent:**
   - Obtaining informed consent from parents or legal guardians for medical procedures, treatments, and research involving pediatric patients.
3. **End-of-Life Decisions:**
   - Navigating ethical dilemmas related to end-of-life care, including decisions about withdrawing or withholding life-sustaining treatments.
4. **Truth-Telling and Age-Appropriate Communication:**
   - Communicating medical information truthfully to pediatric patients while considering their developmental stage and ability to comprehend.
5. **Confidentiality and Privacy:**
   - Maintaining confidentiality and privacy while also involving parents or guardians in discussions about a child's health, particularly in cases of sensitive issues.
6. **Cultural Competence and Respect:**
   - Respecting and integrating cultural beliefs and

practices into care while ensuring the child's best interests are prioritized.

7. **Resource Allocation:**
    ○ Ethical considerations in situations where resources are limited, necessitating decisions about the allocation of care and treatments.

8. **Advocacy for Vulnerable Populations:**
    ○ Advocating for the rights and well-being of vulnerable pediatric populations, such as children with disabilities, chronic illnesses, or those in disadvantaged communities.

9. **Research Involving Children:**
    ○ Ensuring ethical conduct in pediatric research, including obtaining assent from children and informed consent from parents or guardians.

10. **Emergencies and Critical Care:**
    ○ Balancing the need for rapid decision-making in emergencies with ethical considerations, such as resuscitation efforts and the use of life-saving interventions.

Legal Issues:

1. **Consent and Assent:**
    ○ Adhering to legal requirements for obtaining consent from parents or guardians for medical interventions and obtaining assent from children when applicable.

2. **Child Abuse Reporting:**
    ○ Fulfilling legal obligations to report suspected cases of child abuse or neglect to appropriate authorities.

3. **Privacy Laws (HIPAA):**
    ○ Complying with privacy laws, such as the Health

Insurance Portability and Accountability Act (HIPAA), to protect the confidentiality of patient information.

4. **Guardianship and Custody Issues:**
   - Navigating legal complexities related to guardianship and custody, especially in cases where there may be disputes among parents or caregivers.

5. **Medical Records Documentation:**
   - Ensuring accurate and complete documentation of patient care in medical records, adhering to legal standards.

6. **Malpractice and Negligence:**
   - Mitigating the risk of legal actions related to malpractice or negligence by providing competent and standard-of-care nursing practice.

7. **Scope of Practice:**
   - Working within the legal scope of practice for pediatric nursing, understanding and following state regulations and licensure requirements.

8. **Drug Administration and Medication Errors:**
   - Adhering to legal standards in drug administration and responding appropriately to medication errors to ensure patient safety.

9. **School Nursing Laws:**
   - Understanding and complying with laws related to school nursing, including medication administration, immunization compliance, and health screenings.

10. **Advance Directives for Children:**
    - Addressing legal considerations related to advance directives for children, especially in cases where a child has a chronic illness or life-limiting condition.

Strategies for Addressing Ethical and Legal Issues:

1. **Ethics Committees:**
   - Utilizing ethics committees within healthcare institutions to provide guidance and support in navigating complex ethical issues.
2. **Education and Training:**
   - Ensuring ongoing education and training for pediatric nurses on ethical principles, legal requirements, and cultural competence.
3. **Open Communication:**
   - Encouraging open communication between healthcare providers, patients, and families to address concerns, clarify expectations, and make collaborative decisions.
4. **Collaboration with Legal Advisors:**
   - Collaborating with legal advisors within healthcare institutions to seek guidance on legal issues and risk management.
5. **Documentation:**
   - Maintaining accurate and detailed documentation of patient care, including informed consent discussions and any deviations from standard practice.
6. **Patient and Family Advocacy:**
   - Advocating for the rights and best interests of pediatric patients and their families, acting as their liaison within the healthcare system.
7. **Continuous Quality Improvement:**
   - Participating in continuous quality improvement initiatives to enhance patient care, prevent errors, and address system-level issues.
8. **Cultural Competence Training:**

- ◦ Providing ongoing training on cultural competence to enhance nurses' ability to navigate diverse cultural perspectives ethically.
9. **Collaboration with Interdisciplinary Teams:**
   - ◦ Collaborating with interdisciplinary teams, including ethics committees, legal advisors, social workers, and child life specialists, to address multifaceted ethical and legal issues.
10. **Advocacy for Policy Changes:**
    - ◦ Participating in advocacy efforts to influence policies and laws that impact pediatric nursing practice, patient care, and healthcare outcomes.

Ethical and legal considerations are integral components of pediatric nursing practice. By staying informed, fostering open communication, and collaborating with interdisciplinary teams, pediatric nurses can navigate these complex issues and provide high-quality, patient-centered care to children and their families.

Milton Keynes UK
Ingram Content Group UK Ltd.
UKHW020026141223
434291UK00015B/859